◄§ An Illustrated History of the Herbals ੪►

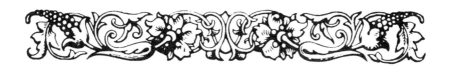

AN ILLUSTRATED

HISTORY OF THE

HERBALS

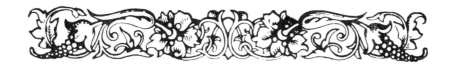

FRANK J. ANDERSON

NEW YORK ✳ COLUMBIA UNIVERSITY PRESS

Library of Congress Cataloging in Publication Data

Anderson, Frank J   1912–
An illustrated history of the herbals.

Bibliography: p.
1. Botany, Medical—History—Sources.
2. Herbs—History—Sources.   3. Botanical literature.
4. Botany—History—Sources.   I. Title.   II. Title: Herbals.
QK99.A1A5   582   77-8821
ISBN 0-231-04002-4

Columbia University Press
New York—Guildford, Surrey

To my wife

KATHLEEN

*whose encouragement, criticism, and
assistance made this book possible.*

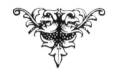

◆§ ACKNOWLEDGMENTS ৯◆

As is the case with everyone who has ever written a book, I have incurred a debt of gratitude to many individuals along the way and would like to take this opportunity to express my thanks. First of all I want to thank the Rare Book Division of the New York Public Library, and its Photo Division, for supplying the illustration to the chapter on Bartholomaeus Anglicus. Thanks also go to the New York Horticultural Society and their Librarian, Miss Barbara Heinen, for permission to reproduce pages from one of the great herbal rarities, *The Herbal of Apuleius.* Thanks are likewise due to Miss Claudia Beldengreen and Miss Gabrielle Beasley, who performed all the necessary photographic services leading to the illustration of this work. And most notably I am indebted to the Library of the New York Botanical Garden and its staff, since the superb collection of herbals at that institution formed the foundation of this book. I am particularly grateful to the successive curators of that library, Mr. John Reed (presently Director of Educational Services at NYBG), and to the present Administrative Librarian, Mr. Charles R. Long, both of whom granted me full access to all material that I needed.

✦§ CONTENTS §✦

Illustrations *xi*

Introduction *1*

1 The *De Materia Medica* of Dioscorides *7*

2 Pliny's *Naturalis Historia* *16*

3 The *Herbal of Apuleius* *23*

4 The *De Viribus Herbarum* of Macer Floridus *30*

5 Mesue the Younger, *Opera Quae Extant Omnia;*
   Serapion the Younger, *Liber Serapionis Aggregatus* *36*

6 The *Circa Instans* of Matthaeus Platearius *45*

7 The *Physica* of Hildegarde of Bingen *51*

8 Bartholomaeus Anglicus *De Proprietatibus Rerum* *59*

9 The *Opus Ruralium Commodorum* of Pietro Crescenzi *66*

10 Conrad von Megenberg's *Buch der Natur* *73*

11 Peter Schoeffer's *Herbarius Latinus* *82*

12 Peter Schoeffer's *Der Gart* *89*

13 *Arbolayre,* or *Le Grant Herbier* *98*

14 Jacob Meydenbach's *Hortus Sanitatis* *106*

15 *Das Buch zu Distillieren* of Hieronymus Brunschwig *113*

16 The *Herbarum Vivae Eicones* of Otto Brunfels *121*

17 The *Kreüter Buch* of Hieronymus Bock *130*

18 The *De Historia Stirpium* of Leonhart Fuchs *137*

19 The *New Herball* of William Turner *148*

20 The *Kreütterbuch* of Adam Lonitzer *156*

21 The *Commentarii* of Pier Andrea Mattioli *163*

22 The *Crüÿdeboeck* of Rembert Dodoens *173*

23 Thurneisser's *Historia* *181*

24 The *Herbario Nuovo* of Castore Durante *187*

25 The *Phytognomonica* of Giambattista Porta *193*

26 The *Coloquios* of Garcia da Orta, and the *Dos Libros* of Nicolas Monardes *201*

27 The *Phytobasanos* of Fabio Colonna *210*

28 The *Herball* of John Gerard *218*

29 Parkinson's *Theatrum Botanicum* *227*

30 The *Rerum Medicarum* of Francisco Hernandez *235*

Glossary *245*
Bibliography *251*
Index *259*

ILLUSTRATIONS

1. Four cucurbits   9
2. Draco marinus   11
3. Three nasturtiums   12
4. Two nymphaeas   13
5. The Astronomer   18
6. North and south winds   19
7. Book XII, Trees   20
8. Book VIII, Animals   21
9. Aristolochia   25
10. Verbena   27
11. Nepite (Catnip)   28
12. Maurella (*Atropa belladonna*)   31
13. Pulegium (Pennyroyal)   31
14. Portrait of Macer   33
15. Scammony   38
16. Rose   38
17. Page of text, Serapion, 1473 ed.   41
18. Title page, Serapion, 1525 ed.   43
19. Incipit *Circa instans*, 1497 ed.   47
20. Cosmas and Damian   53
21. Physicians consulting   54
22. Wound Man   55
23. Title page of *De proprietatibus rerum* (detail)   61
24. Rosemary   68
25. Pomegranate   68
26. Borage   69
27. Creation and Expulsion of Man   71
28. Plants   75
29. Monsters   76
30. The Heavens   78
31. Bees, Insects, Worms   79

32. Sea Wonders *80*
33. Coriander *83*
34. Madder *84*
35. Arnaldus and Avicenna *85*
36. Frontispiece of *Der Gart* *91*
37. Musk Deer *93*
38. Cannabis *94*
39. Viola *95*
40. Columbine *95*
41. Title page of *Le Grant Herbier* *100*
42. Plantain *102*
43. Fuller's teasle *102*
44. Cepe (Onion) *103*
45. Caladrius *108*
46. Pistris *108*
47. Physician in apothecary shop *110*
48. Title page of *Buch zu Distillieren* *115*
49. Sick-bed *116*
50. Stills and furnaces *118*
51. Title page of Brunfels' herbal *123*
52. Geranium *124*
53. Herba Paralysis *125*
54. Hepatica *126*
55. Sanicle (All Heal) *127*
56. Buxbaum *131*
57. Portrait of Bock *133*
58. Mulberry; Pyramus and Thisbe *135*
59. Salvia (Sage) *139*
60. Small portrait of Fuchs *140*
61. *Cucumis turcicus* *141*
62. Full-length portrait of Fuchs *142*
63. Lupulus (Hops) *143*
64. Four cucurbits *144*
65. Cuckoo pynt *150*
66. Anagyris (text and decorative initial) *151*
67. Bittersweet *153*

68. Kebuli (text and decorative initial) *154*

69. Adam and Eve and the Tree *158*

70. Medicine and herbs *159*

71. Mining scene *160*

72. Barnyard *161*

73. Portrait of Mattioli *165*

74. Almonds *166*

75. Garden Nightshade *167*

76. Hazelnuts *169*

77. Psyllium *170*

78. Portrait of Dodoens *175*

79. Title page of *A Nievve Herball* *176*

80. Portrait of Thurneisser *183*

81. Umbellifer *184*

82. Astrological chart *185*

83. Six plants from the *Herbario Nuovo* *188*

84. Camphora *189*

85. Portrait of Durante *190*

86. Wild olive *191*

87. Title page of Porta's *Phytognomonica* *195*

88. Heart plants *196*

89. Plants for scaly diseases *197*

90. Portrait of Porta *198*

91. Portrait of Monardes *203*

92. Guaiacum *204*

93. Bangue (Cannabis) *205*

94. Pepper *207*

95. Astragalus *212*

96. Phu *213*

97. Tragium (Goat's Beard) *214*

98. Phyteuma *215*

99. Dragon Tree *220*

100. Portrait of Gerard *221*

101. Round-rooted Crowfoot *222*

102. Cloves *223*

103. Mistletoe *224*

104. Portrait of Parkinson   229
105. Title page of *Theatrum Botanicum*   231
106. Title page of *Paradisi in Sole*   233
107. Taurus Mexicanus   237
108. Opuntia   238
109. Title page of *Rerum Medicarum*   241
110. Metl   242

❦ An Illustrated History of the Herbals ❧

Introduction

A S A C L A S S, herbals are among the most fascinating of
books but also among the least familiar, except to a relatively small number of scholars. This can be attributed to
their great rarity, and to the fact that they were generally
written either in Latin or in equally difficult medieval German, French, or English. But since their pages hold so much
interesting material in a variety of areas, it is regrettable that
they are so seldom made available to informed laymen. This
illustrated survey of herbals is presented as a partial remedy
to that situation.

In the pages that follow there are carefully selected pictures from the herbals themselves, together with background information about each work. These brief histories
or resumés present facts about each book, its author, its
place among other herbals, and other matters of special significance. Essentially this is a herbal sampler in which the
unique character and flavor of each book is conveyed to the
reader, while providing him with a comprehensive view of
the development of herbal literature.

By definition, a "herbal" is a book that is descriptive of
plants. It is, however, a great deal more than that. For one

thing, herbals generally concern themselves mostly with plants that have medicinal properties, and they usually include some information as to how to identify them, extract their useful properties, and then apply them to cure certain disorders, wounds, and diseases. But it would be erroneous to give the impression that herbals are only about plants, for they draw their medicaments from other sources as well. In fact, one of the most comprehensive of the herbals, the *Hortus sanitatis,* is something of a medieval natural history, and describes the animal and mineral kingdoms as well as the vegetable one.

The term "herbal" did not come into use until the beginning of the sixteenth century, but works of a medico-botanical nature had been produced since the dawn of civilization. The earliest records from Egypt, Sumer, and China all provide examples of such works, and it is evident from their complexity and range that they reflect a tradition that was old long before the invention of writing. The antiquity of these early works is indicated by their claims that herbs were made from the flesh of the gods, who also instructed men in their proper use.

Among the initial herbals was the *Papyrus Ebers* which, although its earliest copy dates from about 1550 B.C., contains material originally written from five to twenty centuries before. It is the most complete and extensive of the ancient herbals that have survived. There is also a tablet from Sumer, dating from about 3000 B.C., that lists about a dozen prescriptions from some physician's repertoire of cures. Restricted to relatively few ingredients such as cassia, thyme, figs, milk, salt, and saltpetre, the limited pharmacopeia was more versatile than might appear at first sight, for from it could be made laxatives, detergents, antiseptics, salves, filtrates, and astringents. And in China, probably about 2700 B.C., the legendary Emperor Shen Nung composed the Pen T'sao Ching, containing about a hundred herbal remedies.

Nothing in the west approaches such antiquity. According to records, the first herbal in Greece was written in the third century B.C. by Diocles of Carystus, but nothing remains of the herbal itself. Only a few fragments of the next major herbal, that of Crateuas, survive from the first century B.C. It was not until the first century of the Christian era that a herbal was composed which is still extant. It is a work by Pedanios Dioscorides of Anazarba called *De materia medica*, and it came into being sometime about A.D. 65. A product of the classical world of Greece and Rome, it is the single most influential herbal ever written. For over 1,500 years it was the final authority on pharmacy, and retained that position even as late as the nineteenth century in Turkey and Spain.

Because Dioscorides provided the foundation of all herbal literature that was to develop from his day forward, it is with his work that this survey will begin. Proceeding from that point all of the subsequent herbals will be listed and discussed in the chronological order of their composition. The illustrations and samples of text, however, will be chosen from the printed editions that began to be published in the fifteenth century. The first of these was the *Historia naturalis* of Caius Plinius Secundus (Pliny), which appeared in Venice in 1469 from the press of Johannes Spira, some nine years before Dioscorides was set in type.

The decision to present a survey based on the printed versions of the herbals, rather than on manuscript copies, was made for several reasons. Most herbal literature was created after the invention of printing, and very few manuscripts of some of the early herbals have survived. For some of them it is even doubtful if any manuscript, other than a working copy for the printer, ever existed. Other problems with manuscripts are their frequent lack of illustration, and the great variation that exists among them because of scribal errors. With the advent of printing a standard text became possible for the first time, and scholars could cite passages with certainty as to both the wording and location of a particular paragraph and page. That was an attainment rarely if ever reached in the manuscript era simply because of the numerous variations introduced by page sizes, the calligraphic practices of individual scribes, and the scribes' uneven accuracy in matters of hearing, reading, and spelling.

A further deciding factor in favor of the printed herbals is that their production is intimately related to the history of printing itself. Herbal works, because they were of considerable interest to the wealthy physicians and merchants, tended to be prime candidates for publication. In herbal incunabula (books printed before 1501) are to be found some of the finest examples of early printing. The Roman type designed for Spira's edition of Pliny is one instance. Printing, since it originated in Germany, was powerfully influenced by the Gothic script. Not until it spread to Italy, where the Carolingian book-hand and chancery script were still the models of legibility, did the art of printing lose the somewhat cramped, heavy, and slightly illegible type faces of the Gothic style. Florentine and Venetian illustration and ornamentation were of enormous influence on the subsequent design and appearance of books. In the herbals, also, the rapid development of the art of illustration from the fifteenth through the seventeenth centuries is clearly visible. Splendid specimens of etching (introduced to the book printer's repertoire by a herbal), engraving, and register are to be found, along with examples of the major type faces, presses, and printers of Europe. Aldus, Fust and Schoeffer, Verard, Plantin, and many others are represented in herbal printing, as are such notable artists and engravers as Hans von Weiditz and Crispin van de Passe.

The virtues of herbals are not limited to their medical and botanical content nor to their place in the history of printing. They also contain material for the philologist (since many early vernacular dialects occur in them), the social historian (who can often find information about neglected procedures and exotic sources of supply), and the folklorist (who can practically reconstruct the *Physiologus* from herbal tracts on animals, and trace superstitious practices to their origins in Rome, Greece, and the Orient). Because they are such rich repositories of learning, lore, history, and exploration (many medicaments came from the Far East and the New World), they present a close-up view of the manners and beliefs of the classical and medieval worlds and provide us with a picture of the transition from the era of empiricism and superstition to the era of science. Those who already know and enjoy something of the special atmosphere and flavor of the herbals will need no invitation to renew their acquaintanceship. And it is the hope of this book that those who are encountering herbals for the first time will be encouraged to seek still further and deeper.

The *De Materia Medica* of Dioscorides

LMOST any schoolboy can tell you that Homer wrote the *Iliad,* and Euclid the *Elements of Geometry,* but should you inquire about Dioscorides you are likely to get a long silence. Despite the relative neglect that has only lately obscured his name, Dioscorides is of the first importance to medicine and the plant sciences. His writings were the supreme, unarguable authority on medicinal substances for over 1,500 years, and because of the problems of plant identification that they posed, science was led to the development of modern botany.

Dioscorides' only surviving work is his *De materia medica,* chiefly known today to an ever dwindling number of botanists and physicians, but once the fountainhead of all the European herbals. Such magic and charisma were attached to his name that many manuscripts bearing no relation to his were eventually attributed to him. The modern science of pharmacology can be traced back to Dioscorides' efforts to systematize man's knowledge of the materials of

medicine. The highly practical nature of his text is precisely
what gave it precedence over the more philosophical work
of Theophrastus, who was more interested in plants themselves than in what they could or couldn't do for man. One
can scarcely blame those who gave the authority to Dioscorides, for in his pages they could find relief from pain,
whereas Theophrastus might very well engage them in a
serene and lengthy discussion of the form, structure, and
reproductive processes of some particular plant. Dioscorides
preferred a pragmatic approach to plants and vegetable substances: if a plant was not useful it was simply disregarded.

Of Dioscorides himself very little is known. He
flourished about A.D. 60, at which time it is likely that he
wrote the *Materia medica* and dedicated it to his friend and
fellow physician, Areius. He speaks of having travelled
widely, having led a soldier's life, his lifelong interest in the
matter of medicinal substances, and Areius having urged
him to bring together all that he had learned about that subject. Dioscorides freely admits that his work is a compilation, but his text is frequently augmented by his own observations and experience. From the mention of Areius and a
friend of his, one Licinius Bassus, it would appear that
Dioscorides lived and wrote in the time of Nero. He may
even have served in Nero's armies, or those of Caligula or
Claudius, who immediately preceded Nero. The name by
which he was known to his contemporaries, Pedanius Dioscorides of Anazarba (a small town near Tarsus), informs us
that he was a Cilician, and that his native language, in
which his books were written, was Greek. This was the case
with most physicians of his era. Beyond these few facts,
which come from the introduction to Dioscorides' *Materia
medica*, all else is speculation. The Greek text of the *Materia
medica* was translated into Syriac when pagan Greek scholars
fled eastward after Constantine's conquest of Byzantium.
Later it was translated into Arabic and Persian, and became
an important element in the medical knowledge of the Mos-

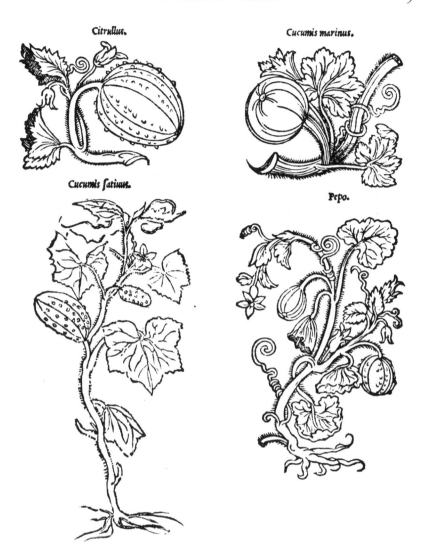

Citrullus.

Cucumis marinus.

Cucumis satiuus.

Pepo.

FIGURE 1. Four cucurbits. These four specimens of the gourd family originally appeared in Fuchs's *Historia Stirpium,* from which they were adapted
by Christian Egenolph of Frankfort for his 1543 and 1549 editions of Dioscorides. Thieving plagiarist that he was, Egenolph still gave value to his
public, for he combined Jean Ruelle's excellent translation with reduced
woodcuts from Fuchs's herbal. The 1549 edition improved the bargain
even further by adding the famous commentaries by Valerius, Eurich
Cordus, and Conrad Gesner. (From Dioscorides' *De Materia Medica.*
Frankfort am Main, Egenolph, 1549. Original size 5 1/8" wide × 6 7/8" high.)

lem world. In the West it was translated into Latin where, in various forms, it survived until the Renaissance. From that time onward it appeared (generally with ample commentaries) in German, French, English, Italian, Spanish, and Bohemian. Other herbals were developed out of it, and it was cited frequently in many well-known works such as *Der Gart*, the *Hortus sanitatis* and the *Herbarius latinus*. For that matter it was still being quoted in the 1720 edition of Quincy's *Pharmacopeia officinalis* and, it is said, remained the botanical standard in nineteenth-century Spain and Turkey. Even as late as 1970, *El Dioscorides Renovado* was issued in Barcelona.

The original Greek manuscript is no longer extant, and the oldest known manuscript is incorporated in the Juliana Anicia Codex of c. A.D. 512. Now preserved in the Austrian National Library at Vienna, where it is Codex Vindobonensis Med. Gr.I, it was discovered in 1562 in Turkey by the Ambassador from the Holy Roman Empire, a Flemish antiquarian named Ogier Busbecq. It was then in the possession of the son of Hamon, former physician to the Sultan Suleiman the Great, who wanted 100 ducats for it. Sometime between then and 1569, when it entered Vienna and the library of Maximilian, the sum was paid, but when and by whom nobody knows.

The codex is a direct link with the world of classical antiquity, for it contains illustrations that are said to be modelled on those of Crateuas, a Greek herbalist and artist of the first century B.C. It is quite possible that his illuminated manuscript may have survived down to the Byzantium of the sixth century A.D., or that faithful copies of it still existed at that time. In any case the plants are depicted with a greater degree of skill than was elsewhere evident in the Byzantine art of that era, which was very little concerned with subjects of nature, preferring theological and hieratic themes. The codex, as a matter of fact, was the outgrowth of religious activity, for it was a birthday gift from the people

Draco marinus. Caput XII.

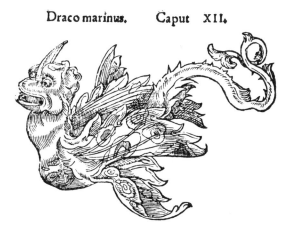

FIGURE 2. Draco marinus. Somewhat Chinese or Javanese in style, this creature is a most improbable cross between a reptile, a butterfly, a fantailed goldfish, and a one-horned ape. It is supposed to represent a sea-dragon, of which Dioscorides has only this to say: "being opened and so applied it is a cure for wounds made by its barbs." Although transformed into a legendary monster this dragon may very well have been based on the stingray, which could inflict a painful wound. (From Dioscorides' *De Materia Medica*. Frankfort am Main, Egenolph, 1549. Original size 4 ⅛" wide × 3 ⅛" high.)

of Honoratae, a suburb of Byzantium, where Juliana Anicia had arranged for the construction and decoration of a church to the martyr, Polyeuktos. She was of a wealthy and aristocratic line. Her father, Anicius Olybrius, had been Emperor of the West for a brief period before his death in A.D. 472.

The text of the Juliana Anicia codex follows a different order from the plan set forth by Dioscorides himself. In the introduction to his *Materia medica* he complains that some earlier writers had done a disservice to physicians by classifying medicines alphabetically, thereby separating some that were closely related, and making it more difficult to learn their particular qualities and operations. The Juliana Anicia Codex is, however, set in just such an alphabetical

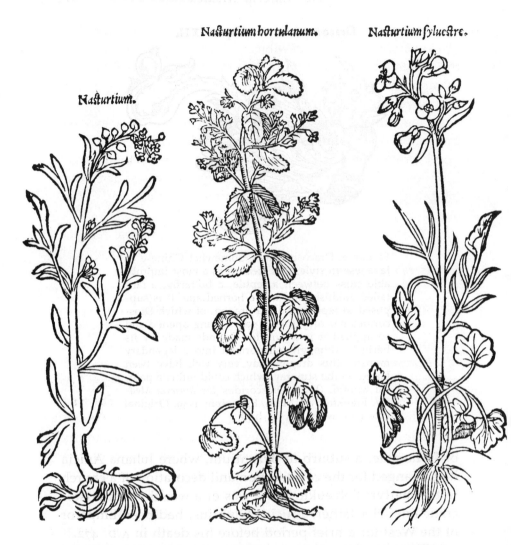

Nasturtium.

Nasturtium hortulanum.

Nasturtium sylucstre.

FIGURE 3. Three nasturtiums. The nasturtium (nose-twister) of Dioscorides was not the ornamental flower so often found in gardens, but a
kind of cress. In earlier times its seed was prescribed for driving out
worms, or to act as an aphrodisiac, and even to procure an abortion. It
was also reputed to stop hair from falling out, to cleanse impetigo and
spotty skins, and, when mixed with flour and vinegar, to relieve sciatica.
All in all, a versatile plant if it really lived up to its billing. (From Dioscorides' *De Materia Medica*. Frankfort am Main, Egenolph, 1549. Original
size 5 ¹/₄" wide × 5 ¹/₂" high.)

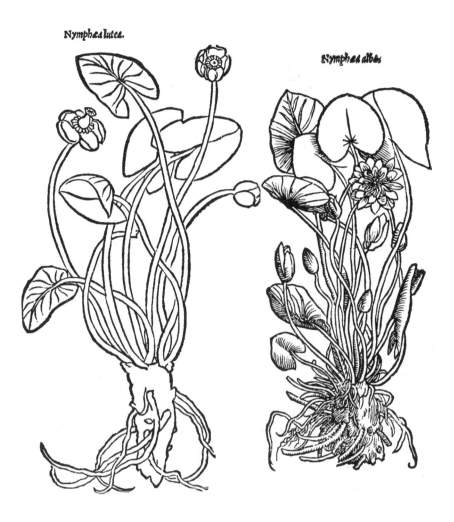

FIGURE 4. Two nymphaeas. The nymphaea of Dioscorides is probably the
European white water-lily (*Nymphaea alba*) rather than the closely related
Egyptian lotus, which is not a true lotus at all despite its name. Besides
prescribing it for ailments of the spleen and for dysentery, Dioscorides
recommended that it be mixed with pitch so as to stop falling hair. It is
certain that if the nymphaea failed, the pitch could be counted upon.
Dioscorides also used it to allay sexual dreams, and to reduce desire.
(From Dioscorides' *De Materia Medica*. Frankfort am Main, Egenolph,
1549. Original size 5 ¹/₂" wide × 6 ¹/₈" high.)

order, whereas Dioscorides had divided his work into five separate books, each of which grouped medicines by form and origin rather than by botanical, zoological, or mineralogical systems. Book I treated of aromatics, oils, ointments, and trees; Book II was on living creatures, milk and dairy produce, cereals, and sharp herbs; Book III discussed roots, juices, herbs, and seeds; Book IV took up those roots and herbs not spoken of elsewhere; and Book V was concerned with wines and metallic ores. It is difficult, however, to discern any advantage to the Dioscoridean distribution of herbs, for those that are used for diuretics, cathartics, emetics, or other purposes are mixed together in random order.

In Europe the nonalphabetical versions of Dioscorides prevailed, though most herbals were arranged quite differently. Numerous Latin manuscripts circulated there until Greek scholars, fleeing westward from the Turks after the fall of Constantinople, brought Greek, Arabic, and Hebrew translations with them, which western scholars used for comparison, emendation, and correction. This infusion of knowledge from the east closely coincided with the invention of printing, and the *Materia medica* was soon available in many editions.

With the arrival of standardized and critical texts there began a series of botanical discussions and investigations that led to the separation of botany from medicine (to which it had been tied for centuries), and then to its subsequent development as an independent science. Many of the Renaissance botanists, situated in Germany, Flanders, England, and France, had attempted to reconcile the plants Dioscorides described with their own local flora. The results were discouraging until they were finally led into the realization that different regions produced different species. With that now obvious conclusion, which imperfect communication had retarded until then, there came the beginning of botanical science. Out of error truth eventually emerged, and Dioscorides' *Materia medica* was the instrument through which it prevailed. A foundation stone in the natural sciences, it is fully deserving of all the importance scholars have attached to it, and it should be granted continued recognition in the future.

BIBLIGRAPHIC NOTES

Original manuscript of c. A.D. 60 not extant.

Oldest manuscript in the Codex Juliana Anicia of c. A.D. 512, now listed as Codex Vindobonensis Med. Gr. 1 in the National Library, Vienna, Austria.

1st edition in Latin: 1478 at Colle, Tuscany, Italy, by Johannem Allemanum de Medemblick.

1st edition in Greek: 1504, Venice, by Aldus Manutius.

1st illustrated edition: 1543 at Frankfort, by Christian Egenolph. Contains 595 woodcuts.

English translation by John Goodyer in 1655, edited by Robert T. Gunther; first printed in 1933, Hafner Publishing Co., London and New York. Remains in print as of 1977.

A facsimile of the Codex Juliana Anicia is also available in full color and with scholarly comment and notes (in German) from the National Library at Vienna, Austria, printed in 1970 by Akademische Druck und Verlagsanstalt, Graz, Austria.

❧ 2 ❧

Pliny's *Naturalis Historia*

E W works have been the subject of as much praise and damnation as Pliny's *Naturalis Historia*. Though lauded by the ancient and medieval worlds, its reputation undeservedly declined once men entered the age of science and thought they knew more than they did. The mountain of facts Pliny presented was somehow ignored, while his minor sins in the realm of fantasy were loudly decried. Fiction and fable, however, as we are finally beginning to realize, very often turn out to be fact in disguise. Quite recently that seafaring scientist, Jacques Cousteau, filmed a sequence in the Indian Ocean which substantiated a tale of Pliny's that scholars had laughed at for centuries. The story was that dolphins were known to drive schools of fish into the shallows where men stood waiting with nets to catch them. Whether or not the dolphins deserve credit for acting in partnership with man, the fact remains that the whole sequence of events happened just as Pliny said it had.

For some strange reason a kind of intellectual myopia has affected our view of Pliny's masterwork in more ways than one. Even the title that Pliny himself bestowed upon it,

Naturalis Historia, has been reversed into *Historia Naturalis,* a minor difference, true enough, and of no importance in Latin, but one that introduces an inconsistency which alters the order of alphabetical listings in bibliographic works already overloaded with complexities. Pliny is also often accused of a lack of critical selection, but seldom is there a word of gratitude for those works his unselective stylus has preserved for us, works that otherwise would have disappeared. Thanks to Pliny, large portions of the writings of two of the ancient herbalists, Diocles and Crateuas, still survive.

To gather his wide range of material Pliny had to make himself familiar with some 2,000 manuscripts. This was no small task in itself, for they were in the awkward form of thousands of scrolls. Out of that enormous mass of data he extracted a sizable body of facts and observations, as he himself tells us in Book I of his *Natural History,* which is the table of contents to the whole work. There he lists 33,727 items, carefully totalling them up for all but three of the 36 remaining books. He was equally careful about crediting his sources, appending the names of the authors he consulted in the creation of every separate book. In his prefatory remarks, Pliny estimated that he used only 100 authors, but over 400 are actually tabulated in his text. It is plain that he was conservative in such estimates, modestly claiming only 20,000 facts for the *Natural History* when, by actual count, it contained well over 33,000. That he included myths, superstitions, and tall tales is genuinely to the good, for they give us insight into the Roman world view.

To copy out such a voluminous manuscript was an enormous task, and only the very wealthy could afford to commission such a work. It often was a communal endeavor in the medieval monasteries. As Ernst Meyer, the great historian of botany, once suggested, it was probably the size and cost of the *Naturalis Historia* that kept it intact during the many dangerous times it passed through, since men generally take good care of anything that is unusually expensive. Despite its length Pliny's work was often copied, sometimes in abridged versions. About 200 more or less complete manuscripts are known, the oldest of which dates to around the 10th century A.D. Establishing dates and provenance for such manuscripts is notoriously difficult and subject to error.

Most important from the standpoint of the herbalist were Pliny's books on trees, plants, and medicaments (Books XII–XXVII). Out of his 37 books (actually lengthy chapters by today's standards) 16 are concerned with plants,

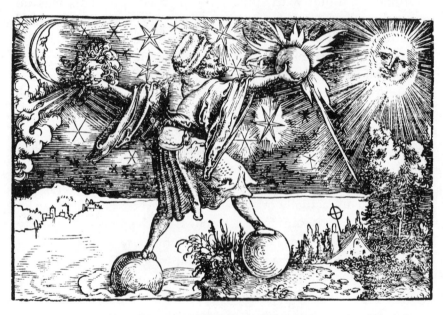

FIGURE 5. The Astronomer. Striding his globes beneath a star-studded sky bounded on either side by the sun and moon, the astronomer holds the wind and catches the fire of the sun. The design, created by Hans von Weiditz, was used in a 1582 edition of Pliny, and captures the majesty of his opening book on the universe. (From Pliny's *Historia naturalis.* Frankfort am Main, Feyerabend, 1582. Original size 6 3/8″ wide × 3 7/8″ high.)

and 18 with medicines and diseases. There is a certain amount of overlap, for 8 of the plant-based books also discuss medicines obtained from herbs, shrubs, fruits, and trees.

Nowhere does Pliny mention Dioscorides as a source, although the two men were roughly contemporary and frequently made very similar statements about the medicines they described. The answer lies not in plagiarism on the part of either, but in the probability that they consulted a common source, perhaps Diocles, Crateuas or, more likely, Sextius Niger. Both Pliny and Dioscorides were cited time

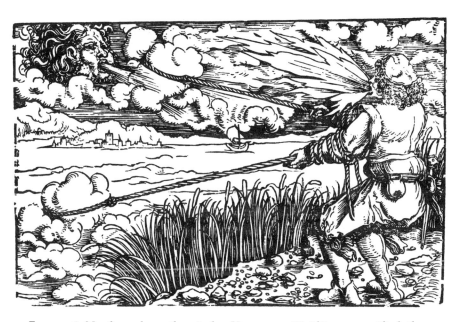

FIGURE 6. North and south winds. Hans von Weiditz personified the winds much as Pliny did, showing the hot South Wind exhaling flame, and hauling on a cloud formed where his breath met the cold moisture from the North. The winds were thought to be an underlying cause of thunder. Breath emerging from the earth was subjected to pressure from the stars, and when further checked in its motion by a cloud it struggled to be released, thunder being the noise when it burst free at last. (From Pliny's *Historia naturalis*. Frankfort am Main, Feyerabend, 1582. Original size 6 $^3/_{16}$″ wide × 3 $^7/_8$″ high.)

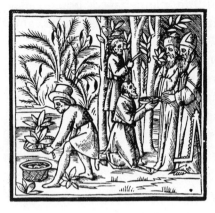

FIGURE 7. Book XII, Trees. Book XII of the *Historia naturalis* is concerned with trees, wherein Pliny mentions that the Romans once considered them to be the temples of the deities. The winter-oak was sacred to Jove, the bay to Apollo, the olive to Minerva, the myrtle to Venus, and the poplar to Hercules. He also tells us that the roots of plane-trees were liberally moistened with wine to make them grow, and the Emperor Caligula once held a banquet in the branches of a great plane-tree at Velletri. (From Pliny's *Historia naturalis*. Venice, M. Sessa, 1513. Original size 3 3/16″ wide × 2 15/16″ high.)

and again in the medieval herbals. Pliny is mentioned 116 times in *Der Gart,* and 264 times in the *Hortus sanitatis.*

Born at Como in A.D. 23, Pliny was educated in Rome toward a career in public service, as had been the family custom. Throughout his life he exemplified the qualities that gave the Romans their supremacy in the ancient world: probity, loyalty, honor, and industry. Pliny had been a captain of the cavalry, spent much time in Germany with the legions, was Governor of Spain, and finally Commander of the Fleet at Misenum. During the reign of Nero he had the wisdom to retire from public life. Customarily he worked until one or two in the morning and was up before dawn to consult with the Emperor Vespasian at the imperial palace. Pliny also practiced law and found time to write six other books besides the *Naturalis Historia,* the only work of his that has not perished. The *Naturalis Historia* was, in fact, the last work that he finished before the fateful day of August 23, A.D. 79, when he died on the beach at Stabiae, a victim of the same eruption of Vesuvius that destroyed Pompeii. Pliny, who was at that time the Commander of the Roman Fleet at Misenum, had been drawn to the area out of curios-

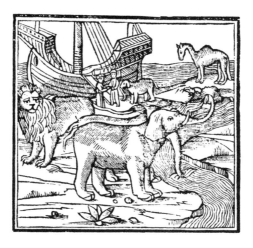

FIGURE 8. Book VIII, Animals. Pliny's Venetian illustrator chose a Noah's Ark theme
to head Book VIII on Animals. The woodcuts are from the 1513 edition by Melchior
Sessa, the first printed version of Pliny to
be illustrated. The elephant, which figures
so prominently in the foreground, is the
first animal discussed by Pliny. He relates
that over 140 of them, among the first to be
seen in Rome, were killed in the Circus
because the Romans of that day, 252 B.C.,
had no other idea of what to do with them.
(From Pliny's *Historia naturalis*. Venice,
M. Sessa, 1513. Original size 3 ³/₁₆" wide ×
2 ¹⁵/₁₆" high.)

ity at the explosion and the plume of dense smoke. He
boarded a light sailing vessel and headed for Stabiae, where
friends of his had a country villa. Once beached he sought
to calm the excited inhabitants and ordered larger vessels
from the fleet to attempt a rescue procedure. The following
morning, high waves prevented him from putting out to
sea, and the rain of ash and pumice grew ever stronger. The
sulphurous fumes overcame him as he rested on the shore,
and when others tried to raise him to his feet they found
that he had died quietly of asphyxiation. With Pliny's un-
timely death at the age of 56 the Roman world, and man-

kind, lost a light of civilization that was only just beginning
to burn at its brightest.

BIBLIOGRAPHIC NOTES

MANUSCRIPT COPIES:

A palimpsest copy, the *Nonantulus* of the 5th or 6th century A.D.,
from the Benedictine Monastery at Nonantula, near Modena.
In Rome (at unnamed location) in 1956.
Earliest manuscript: the *Codex Bamburgensis* of the 10th century
A.D.
Leidensis Vossianus, 11th century A.D. or earlier.
Codex Parisinus latinus 6795, 10th or 11th century A.D.

EARLY EDITIONS:

1st edition by Johann Spira, Venice, 1469.
1st illustrated edition by Melchior Sessa, Venice, 1513.
First commentary and correction of manuscript texts: Hermolaus
Barbarus, *Castigationes Plinianae,* Rome, 1492.

ENGLISH TRANSLATIONS:

Philemon Holland, London, 1601. Selections available.
Bostock and Riley, London, 1855–57. Reprint available.
Loeb Classical Library, London and Cambridge, Mass., 1938–62. In
print.

⋅§ 3 §⋅

The Herbal of Apuleius

HE only certainty about *The Herbal of Apuleius* is that its supposed author never had a hand in writing it. For one thing, there is no agreement about its proper title, as is very often the case with manuscripts, particularly those that originated after the classical world had entered its decline. Some things which the modern world insists upon were of relatively little importance to our ancestors—matters such as the exact measurement of time, explicit written directions for making things, and definitive titles for books.

The Herbal of Apuleius has been known variously as: *De medicaminibus herbarum liber uno; Herbarius Apulei Platonici* (perhaps its most common name); *Herbarium de Sextus Apuleius Barbarus; Herbarium Apuleius Plato;* and *De herbarum virtutibus.* Its author's name, too, has had it variations, including L. Apuleius, Pseudo-Apuleius, Apuleius Barbarus, Apulei Platonici, and others. This has caused some understandable confusion, aggravated by the fact that other works were often attached to the Apuleian herbal. For instance, the work is almost always accompanied by a treatise on betony by a Roman physician, Antonius Musa. Other manuscripts

often found with *The Herbal of Apuleius* are an extract from
Dioscorides termed *Herbae foeminae,* and *De medica-
mentis ex animalibus* of Sexti Platonici Papyrensis. Small
wonder that the early bibliographers were confused as to
just what work they were dealing with.

For some time it was wrongly imagined that Lucius
Apuleius, who wrote the Latin classic *The Golden Ass,*
was identical with the author of the *Herbarius.* In support of
that notion was the fact that Lucius Apuleius was a native of
Madurensis in North Africa (near ancient Carthage), and
was a student of Plato's philosophy. This had some bearing
upon the *Herbal,* for in its text there were included names of
some native North African plants and reptiles, which were
closely associated with Carthage. As for the connection with
Plato, it derived from a depiction of three figures that
formed the first leaf of almost every manuscript of the *Herbal*
that has survived, and the linkage arose from a formidable
combination of ignorance, misunderstanding, and error.
Many of the books of the Graeco-Roman world bore portraits of their authors on the first leaf of the codices (which
were then replacing the less convenient scrolls). *The Herbal
of Apuleius,* following this custom, presented three figures
from mythology, thus giving its contents the authority and
prestige of having emanated from the most ancient, divine,
and credible sources.

One of the personages depicted in the frontispiece was
Chiron the Centaur, who had been granted knowledge of
the medicinal powers of plants by the goddess Diana. Another was Achilles, whom Chiron had instructed in the art
of medicine. The third figure was supposedly that of Apuleius, but was in reality that of Peleus, father of Achilles,
who had placed him under the tutelage of Chiron. Through
ignorance of the classical myths, and misunderstanding of
the Greek characters that set forth the personal names, later
Latin scribes transmuted Peleus into Apuleius. Soon afterwards the figure of Achilles was interpreted as that of

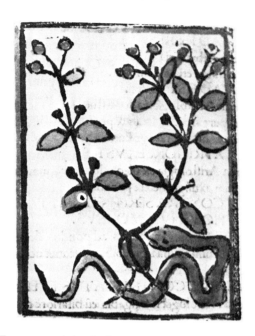

FIGURE 9. Aristolochia. This type of Aristolochia was a different kind from Birthwort, and was used for other purposes, among them driving out demons through fumigation, a method also used to restore a peevish, crying child to a state of laughter and happiness. It cured ulcers, chills, fever, external cancer, and was an antidote for poison. As Apuleius said, no doctor could readily work his cures without it. (From *The Herbal of Apuleius*. Rome, J. Lignamine [1481]. Original size of page 5 ½" wide × 7 ⅞" wide.)

Plato, who *had* to be present if his admirer, Apuleius, was already there. Subsequently Plato's name became still further confused with that of Platearius, a famous twelfth-century physician at Salerno, and error compounded error. Anyone who has closely examined a medieval manuscript can see the enormous potential for error created by numerous contractions, variant spellings, and often dubious (or downright illegible) rendering of the characters of the alphabet.

Even the date of the earliest manuscript of *The Herbal of Apuleius* is not fully agreed upon, nor are the length of the text or the order of the chapters. Claus Nissen claims that Ms. Voss Lat. Q. 9, now preserved at Leyden, is of the 7th century A.D., while Robert T. Gunther, F.W.T. Hunger, and Charles Singer say that it is of the 6th century. The work is variously listed as having 130 or 131 chapters, but at least one manuscript, an Anglo-Saxon translation, has 132. Because the original manuscript went through several recensions, known as the alpha, beta, and gamma versions, it is not possible to determine its authentic length, or the number and order of its chapters. Even the date of the first printed edition is in question, since either its anonymous printer, or its publisher, Philip de Lignamine, did not include the date. The technique used to produce the illustrations is also in doubt. They could have been made from woodcuts, or metal plates, or both. Some illustrations appear to exhibit a granular metallic character, while others seem to show a wood grain. Yet another question is, very simply, what plants are represented in the pictures? Divested of their labels, most of them are impossible to identify.

All in all, *The Herbal of Apuleius* might well be termed "The Puzzles of Apuleius," and at this late date its mysteries are not likely to be solved. From internal evidence it is highly probable that the work was compiled around A.D. 400. It is likely that the original manuscript was written in Greek, and that it drew heavily on Pliny and Dioscorides. There is also a strong likelihood that it was compiled by a layman rather than a physician, for it is remarkably vague about weights, measures, methods of compounding, dosages, etc., all of which physicians were generally careful to state in their prescriptions.

Many elements of popular superstition were carried over into the text of *The Herbal of Apuleius*. Among them were pagan prayers, which supports the argument that the

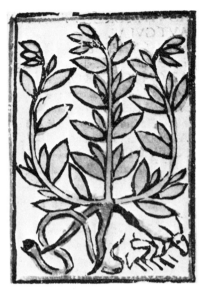

FIGURE 10. Verbena. Apuleius assigned 24 different names to Verbena, and 12 remedial uses. Known to the Anglo-Saxons as Ashthroat, it was applied to ulcers and swellings, and to dog, spider, and snake bites. When eaten it restored digestion and removed bladder-stones and liver ailments. It also made a poultice for wounds and head sores. Apuleius commended its root as a curative amulet, and said that whoever wore the plant was safe from snake-bite. (From *The Herbal of Apuleius*. Rome, J. Lignamine [1481]. Original size of page 5 ¹/₂" wide × 7 ⁷/₈" high.)

work had its origin in the era before Christianity had attained full dominance in the Roman world. One such prayer addressed to "Earth, divine goddess Mother Nature," goes on to plead thus: "Come to me with thy powers, and *howsoever* I may use them, may they have good success, and to *whomsoever* I may give them." The italicized words suggest a reliance on divine favor rather than medical skill. Such prayers were, of course, given a thoroughly Christianized cast in later versions. The Mediterranean plants mentioned

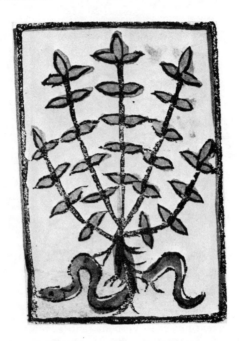

FIGURE 11. Nepite (Catnip). This illustration for
Nepite, Catmint, which has had color added by
hand, clearly shows a granular characteristic
more in keeping with a cast-metal cut than a
woodblock. Other pictures, however, exhibit a
coarse, open grain completely unlike metal, and
it remains uncertain what material was used by
the printer. The snake's presence signifies that
the plant was thought to be antivenomous. (From
The Herbal of Apuleius. Rome, J. Lignamine
[1481]. Original size of page 5 ¹/₂″ wide × 7 ⁷/₈″
high.)

as cures also suffered a few changes, since some of them
were unknown in north and central Europe. The system of
correction commonly adopted was quite simple—it con-
sisted of substituting whatever local plants most resembled
those in the herbal. One monk at St. Gall, compiling an
Apuleius Ms. in the 9th century A.D., left out every plant
that was unknown to him, replacing them with an equal
number of medicinal plants that grew in his locality.

One wonders why such a work had such enormous popularity. Charles Singer characterized it as "a futile work, with its unrecognizable figures and its incomprehensible vocabulary," for it retained plant names from a variety of languages, some of them totally forgotten. And what, indeed, is to be made of a book that recommends placing the root of a peony upon a man to cure him of raging insanity? Equipped with the science of modern medicine, people of the twentieth century can well afford to reject such nonsense. But in an era when classical knowledge had been dispersed, when reliable medical writings were scarcely available, and the medical profession had vanished, when treatment of the sick was entirely left to the charitable but poorly equipped monks, then *The Herbal of Apuleius* was a straw desperately grasped at by despairing men.

BIBLIOGRAPHIC NOTES

Original manuscript c. A.D. 400 no longer extant.
Earliest manuscript: Leyden Ms. Voss Lat. Q. 9 of the 6th century
 A.D.

1st edition: c. 1481 (certainly no later than 1483) by an anonymous
 printer for Philip de Lignamine of Rome.
1st illustrated edition: same as above. *The Herbal of Apuleius* is the
 first fully illustrated herbal ever printed. A botanical illustration in Conrad von Megenburg's *Buch der Natur* preceded it
 by six years, in 1475, but was a single print only, whereas all
 130 plants in Apuleius were figured.

Translation was made into Anglo-Saxon in the 11th century A.D.,
 now preserved at the British Museum as Cotton Ms. Vitellius
 C III, Saec. XI.
The above work is the base for O. Cockayne's English translation
 in *Leechdoms, Wort-cunning and Starcraft of Early England*,
 Rolls Series, London 1864–66, 3 vols. Now out of print.

❧ 4 ❧

The *De Viribus Herbarum* of
Macer Floridus

ESPITE the fact that *The Herbal of Apuleius* represented the lowest level of botany and medicine, it remained one of the most popular medical works of medieval times. It was not until the appearance of Macer's *De viribus herbarum* that it had a serious rival. This work reached every corner of Europe, and was translated from Latin into Polish, French, and English. Only the English translation was completed before the invention of printing. It was done about 1373 by John Lelamar, Master of Hereford School, who does not seem to have had the usual medieval passion for anonymity.

It would be less confusing to be able to say that the author of the *De viribus herbarum* was, indeed, named Macer, as the book's opening line proclaims. Such is not the case, however, for the only known Macer connected with herbal writings is Aemilius Macer, who died in 16 B.C., and he would scarcely have been in a position to cite medieval authorities by name, as is done in *De viribus herbarum*. The chief candidate for authorship is one Odo, Bishop of

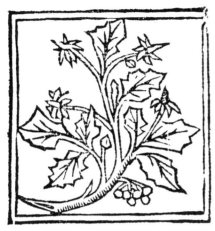 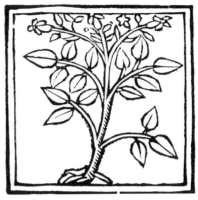

FIGURE 12.   FIGURE 13.

FIGURE 12. Maurella (*Atropa belladonna*). Maurella, or Nightshade (*Atropa belladonna*) was used to cure earaches and headaches, to relieve the burning pain of erysipelas, to stop excessive menstrual bleeding, and for an ailment called aegilops, a swelling in the corner of the eye. This chapter is omitted from some editions of Macer, which are by no means uniform, nor do they follow an invariable order. Supposedly composed of only 77 chapters, there can be as many as 97, 20 of which are spurious. (From Macer's *De virtutibus herbarum*. Baquetier, c. 1510. Original size 2 ¹/₂" wide × 2 ¹/₂" high.)

FIGURE 13. Pulegium (Pennyroyal). *Mentha pulegium* or Pennyroyal had quite a few names—Pudding Grass, Lurk in the Ditch, Pulex, Pulce, and Puce, these last three from its reputation for driving away fleas, pulex being Latin for flea. It was also known as Pulioll-royall, which eventually became Pennyroyal. Macer suggested using it for clearing the chest of phlegm, for nausea and a sick stomach, snake bites, and (when taken with wine) to expel black bile, which was thought to cause melancholy. (From Macer's *De virtutibus herbarum*. Baquetier, c. 1510. Original size 2 ¹/₂" wide × 2 ¹/₂" high.)

Meung, whose name appears on a 12th-century manuscript located in Dresden. The Dresden inscription states "Odonis Magdunensis opusculum de naturis herbarum," or "The Little Work of Otto of Meung, on the Natures of Herbs." Another manuscript of the 13th century, now at Douai, says "De viribus herbarum auctore Odone dicto Macro Floridio," or "Of the Power of Herbs, the author being Odo, called

Macer of the Flowers." There is also Odo Veronensis, who composed a prose abstract of Macer, and Odo Muremundensis of Burgundy, Abbot of Beauprai, whose name turns up on a 14th-century manuscript, although he died in A.D. 1161. And as though that plethora of Odos was not confusing enough, some bibliographers have added yet another possible author, Hugo of Tours. Odo of Meung, however, is most often named, probably more as a bibliographic convenience than anything else.

Although many Mss. of Macer survive there is relatively little discussion of them. David Diringer's *The Illuminated Book* makes no mention of Macer although illustrated manuscripts of it do exist, and Wilfrid Blunt's *Art of Botanical Illustration* also ignores the work. Even in Agnes Arber's excellent *Herbals, Their Origin and Evolution,* only one paragraph is devoted to Macer, describing the first printed edition of 1477, but it is chiefly concerned with a deceptive use of Macer's name in connection with an English herbal.

Macer differs from all other herbals because it is set in Latin verses that describe the medicinal properties of 77 plants. Yet in the first printed edition of 1477, which is also the first herbal ever to be printed, the number of plants is 88, still further compounding a long list of discrepancies. An edition of 1506 lists 86 plants, while some other versions have as many as 97, although 20 of the discussions are deemed to be spurious. Even the name Macer appears variously as Macro, Macron, Macronis, and even Macrobius. He is also referred to either as Philosophi or Floridus, the latter in the printed books from about 1500 onward, and once in manuscript (the Douai of the 13th century A.D.) as Floridio.

Some students of Macer have suggested that he was French, and if Odo of Meung *was* the author, they may be right. Others say that he may have been either a Calabrian

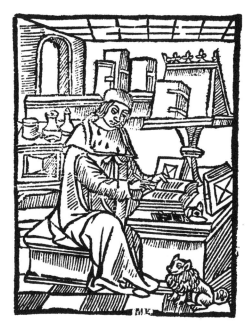

FIGURE 14. Portrait of Macer. One edition of *De Virtutibus herbarum* is headed by what seems to be a portrait of Macer at work on his herbal. In fact it is simply a woodcut that was in the printer's stock, and represents St. Jerome in his study. The lap dog in the lower right-hand corner is what gives the clue, for it is not a Pekinese but a midget-sized version of St. Jerome's companion, the lion whose paw he healed. (From Macer's *De virtutibus herbarum*. Baquetier, c. 1510. Original size 2 ¹/₂″ wide × 4 ¹/₈″ high.)

or a Sicilian, because his language bears strong traces of the Greek that was spoken in both those regions of ancient Magna Graeca. Still others believe either that Macer was a Salernitan, or that the work was written at the School of Salerno. There the first group of lay physicians in Europe was established when the clergy began to relinquish its practice of medicine around A.D. 1000. As with many another enigma from the often vaguely recorded past, it is likely that the debate about Macer's nationality will go on indefinitely.

De viribus herbarum is not an original work except for its use of verse. This feature probably helped it gain acceptance and popularity with physicians, since they could more easily remember metrical lines (Macer's were hexameters) than ordinary prose. The famous poem "Regimen Salernitanum" was widely valued by doctors for this reason.

Most of the material in Macer derives from Pliny. But a Roman physician, Gargilius Martialis, is also represented, as are Galen, Dioscorides, Oribasius, Hippocrates, and a number of other classical writers—23 in all according to Ludwig Choulant, a bibliographer of the history of medicine. The remedies offered in the verses range from those based on sound observation to those that carry strong hints of magic and witchcraft. For instance, Macer recommends "bruising" the flowers and leaves of Senation, or Groundsel (*Senecio vulgaris*), in wine, and applying the mixture to tumors of the rectum and testicles. He also recommends mixing it with frankincense from the frankincense tree, Thure (*Boswellia carteri*), to heal external wounds and relieve pain. These prescriptions are directly from Dioscorides, and may have some basis in fact. But what of the toothache remedy utilizing the same plant? In these verses Macer directs the user to dig up groundsel without using an iron tool, then touch the plant three times to the aching tooth, spitting on the ground each time. Following this ritual the plant is replaced in the soil so it will continue growing, and as long as it lives the tooth will cease to ache. These directives are to be found in Pliny (Book XXV–167) under the plant Erigeron, another name for *Senecio vulgaris,* which is used by both Macer and Dioscorides. The dental remedy, however, is not mentioned by Dioscorides.

Even in Macer's time (either the late 9th century or the early 10th) medicine was still ruled by Roman practices from almost five centuries before.

BIBLIOGRAPHIC NOTES

Original manuscript of *De viribus herbarum* not extant.
Earliest manuscript: *Opus Macri physici de viribus herbarum,* undated but of the 11th century A.D., now at Vienna.

1st edition: 1477 at Naples by Arnold de Bruxella.
1st illustrated edition: 1482 at Milan by Antonius Zarotus of Parma.

∗§ 5 §∗

Mesue the Younger, *Opera Quae Extant Omnia*
Serapion the Younger, *Liber Serapionis Aggregatus*

 HERE are two famous Arabic authors who are not Arabs at all. One is Mesue,[1] who is said to have been a Jacobite Christian of probable Greek origin. The other is Serapion,[2] whose very name proclaims him a Greek, and very likely also a Christian. Neither of these men, as we shall see, may ever have existed, but the Latin west accepted them wholeheartedly and granted their works great influence. These two possibly imaginary authors may well be cited and quoted more often in herbal literature than any of the genuine Arabs save for Avicenna. More importance was attached, in medieval times, to the contents of a book than to the identity of its author, unless of course the author had a

---

[1] Not to be confused with Mesue the Elder, an historic personage of c. A.D. 857.

[2] Not Yahyā ben Sārāfyūn, Serapion Senior, c. A.D. 875.

36

considerable reputation. The casual concern of the age about authorship is plainly seen in the fact that, of the twelve best-selling works among 15th-century incunabula, seven were either anonymous or by apocryphal persons.

Mesue was supposed to have lived at Maradin on the Euphrates, a center for Jacobite Christians, and his dates are given as A.D. 926–1016. Such information as we have about him comes from a mention of him in a book of biographies of Arab physicians and philosophers written by Leo Africanus some 500 years after Mesue's death. Despite the fact that Leo was a Christianized Moslem and a scholar familiar with the events of the Moslem world, his historical work suffered from a lack of accuracy that was common among historians of his day. Unknowingly, Leo may have been writing about an apocryphal person, one that George Sarton calls pseudo-Mesue. To the present date no Arabic manuscript of any of his three medical writings has been found, and Mesue's texts exist only in Latin, Hebrew, and Greek. There is, of course, a possibility that his writings may turn up on some dusty shelf in a remote corner of Islam. There are also grounds for considering Mesue to have been a European author who sought recognition for his work (though not for himself) by giving it an authority borrowed from another time and place.

Mesue's total writings are contained in three books. The first of these, which is known by three different titles, *De medicinis laxativis, De simplicibus,* or *De consolatione,* is concerned with the use of purgatives. It discusses the characteristics of the numerous purges then in use (many courses of treatment at the time began with cleansing out the patient's body), what purge should be chosen, and how it was to be modified in particular cases. The purges are also categorized as gentle, mild, and drastic, and the more potent ones must have acted like tornadoes in the hapless interiors of those who took them.

Mesue's second book was called the *Grabadin* (from the

SCAMONEA.   R O S A.

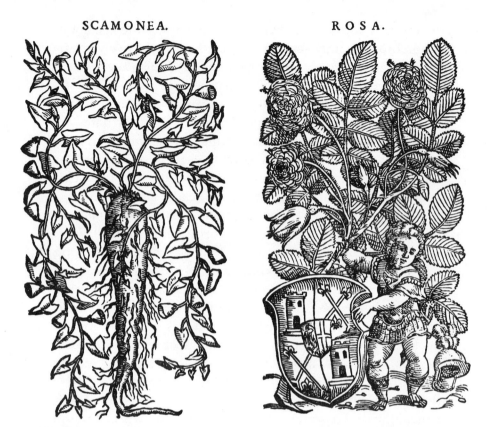

FIGURE 15. Scammony. This is the root of Syrian bindweed (*Convolvulus scammonea*), a drastic purgative possessed of such irritating qualities that its use, particularly in an inflamed intestinal tract, was most dangerous. Since Mesue wrote a good deal on correcting or easing the action of powerful cathartics he had much to say about scammony. Usually the diluted juice of the root was administered according to the patient's strength, but occasionally it was given in combination with other powerful purgatives, with near or fully lethal results. (From Mesue's *Opera omnia*. Venice, V. Valgrisi, 1562. Original size 2 ½" wide × 4 ⅞" high.)

FIGURE 16. Rose. The rose was medicinally important in medieval times, probably as an outgrowth of its extremely agreeable scent. In those days there was a widely held belief that pleasant-smelling plants counteracted the effects of noxious and disease-ridden vapors. By extension, possibly due to the cool, soothing qualities of the petals, the rose was considered useful in treating headache, diseases of the eyes, ears, and gums, hemorrhoids, and erysipelas. It was used to heal wounds, to cure dysentery, and to stop the spitting of blood. (From Mesue's *Opera omnia*. Venice, V. Valgrisi, 1562. Original size 2 ⅝" wide × 4 ⅞" high.)

Arabic term for a formulary, "aqrābādhīn"), and represented an Antidotarium or apothecary's manual. Two medical historians, Garrison and Neuburger, confirm that Mesue's compendium was used everywhere in medieval Europe in the preparation of medicines, and was regarded as "the canon of the apothecary's art . . . held in the highest esteem." The third book attributed to Mesue is his *Liber medicinarum particularum*, an incomplete work on therapeutics.

Who Mesue really was, and where and when he lived, will be debated for years to come. Comparisons of texts now available only in obscure manuscripts may reveal some of the sources of Mesue, as well as those of other dubious writings of the period. For the present, however, Mesue's influence on the development of Western medicine is undeniable, and his name recurs time and again in most of the major herbals. His works were also among the first medical books to be printed. The first edition appeared in Latin in 1471 and was quickly followed by 18 other editions before 1501 (the end of the incunabula period), at least two of which were in Italian.

It may seem odd to deny first place among herbals to Mesue's books, which bear the date of 1471, or to Pliny's *Naturalis Historia*, which was printed in 1469, and reserve the honor instead for Macer's *De virtutibus herbarum* of 1477. The answer lies in the subjects treated, and the manner of their treatment. Pliny's book goes well outside the realm of herbs in many of its sections, and should more accurately be thought of as a general work that contains a herbal among its subjects. The Mesue of 1471 and the Serapion of 1473 both antedate the Macer Floridus of 1477, but their emphasis is more upon pharmacological uses than upon the botanical aspects of medicinal plants. Since medicine, botany, pharmacology, and natural history were not yet separate areas of learning, herbal literature tried to embrace them all. For purposes of more exact definition, works that stress botanical over pharmacological data are more appropriately classed as herbals. It may well be that such a standard is in need of revision in order to ease the burden of bibliographers, but the issue is beyond the scope of this survey, and requires more general agreement about herbals than is presently possible.

The second allegedly Arabic author, whom we know as Serapion, has as vague a background as Mesue. In Serapion's case neither place nor date of birth is known, but he quotes works dating from as late as A.D. 1106. He seems to have been termed a Christian solely on the basis of his supposed Greek origin. No Arabic manuscript of his has ever been found, and no writer in any language speaks of him, cites him, or appears to have known of him until the time of his translators, Simon Januensis and Abraham ben Shemtob (or Abraham Tortuosensis), about 1292.

Simon came from Genoa, hence his name (Januensis). He was physician to Pope Nicholas IV, and was likewise Canon of Rouen. Simon had journeyed to the Aegean islands and to Sicily in order to collect and observe plants, and for almost thirty years he had gathered plant names from travellers from all over the world. Others he had searched out in Greek, Roman, and Arabic works, and in his writings he claims to have used many ancient manuscripts now lost to the modern world. Simon knew the work of Pseudo-Demosthenes and Cassius Felix, both unknown today, two translations of Dioscorides that resemble no oth-

FIGURE 17. Page of text, Serapion, 1473 ed. The first printed edition of Serapion was done in 1473 at Milan by Antonius Zarotus of Parma. His type bears a close resemblance to that of the great Venetian printer Nicolas Jensen, some of whose fonts had been sold just before 1473. The two chapters seen here, on juniper and thyme, still carry many of the symbols and contractions that were characteristic of the manuscripts produced by the medieval scribes. Printing had not yet attained the prestige and desirability of script. (From Serapion. Milan, Zarotus, 1473. Original size of block of type 5 $^7/_8$″ wide × 8 $^7/_8$″ high. With margins added, original page size is 9 $^1/_8$″ wide × 12 $^7/_8$″ high.)

Yſaach.ī tyriaca amomū ē ex rebus
q; inebriāt eſt eni ī ͵ppríetate eius
q̃ febríat & facit dormire.

.IVNIPERVS.

Ab bagar.i.gráum iuníperi.
D.Iuníp̃us ē una ex ſp̃ebus
cipreſi maſchuli & oẽs ſūt quattu
or ſp̃e̅ & ſunt iunipus & habel.i.
ſauia & xeı bın & gar uidelıcet iuni
pus q; nōinat͛ arconas uf archĕcas
eſt ex ea magna & alıa parua & b̃e
fructū & q;dā re pıt cuıus fructus
ē magnus ſicut nabacb & q;dā cu
ius ē puus ſic faba nıſı q̃r ıp̃e ē to
tus rotundus. G.virtus arborıs
prie ē caẛa & ſıcca ī.ııı.gr̃.ſed & calı
dıtas ıpıus fructū ē ſecūdū hoc &
ſiccıtas eıus ē ı prıpıo.ſed ſauına &
ē ılla q; d̃r brachos nō b̃e fructū &
nos ıā dıxıus de ea ſupıus:ſed xer
bın ē ılla q; noıat͛padras b̃e fructū
ſıẛe fructuı cıpreſſı nıſı q̃r ē maıor
eo ſatıs & ē ex xerbın arbor parua
ſpıoſa b̃es fructū ſıẛe fructuı iūi pı
cuıus magnıtudo ē ſıcut grāı mırtı
ſed ē rotōdus & ſero de ıp̃o uenıet
poſtea ı capıtulo de alkıtrā & uırt͛?
xerbın ē caẛa & ſıcca ī.ııı.gr̃.& uır
tus fructus ē tẽpata eq̃lıs adeo q̃
poſıbıle ē q; cōedat͛ nıſı q̃r ſı q̃s co
mederet ex eo mſ̃ıum ınduceret ſo
da & calefaceret corpus & ıuenıret
mordıcatıonē ı ſtō ſuo:Sed gar & ē
ſp̃es pua xerbın mẽoratō eıus uẽı
et ınfra. D.arconas & eſt ıunıpuſ
magna & pua abe calefacıūt & ſub
tılıāt & ͵puocāt urınā & q̃ū ſıt fūı
gatıo cū eıs expellıt uẽeoſa reptılıa
& bẽt fructū cuı͛? qdā repır͛ın ma
gnıtudıe auelãe & qdā ı magıtudıe
fabe nıſı q̃r ē rotūdus & b̃e odorē

---

bonū & ē dulcıs babẽs ī ſe alıq̃tulū
áarıtudīs & nōınát eū arcōas & ca
lefacıt par̃ & eſt ſtıptıcus ac bonus
ſtō & q̃ū ſūıt ex eo ı potu cōfr̃ dolo
rı pectorıs & tuſſı ıſlātıōıbus & tor
tıōıbus & ex̃pellıt uẽena ac ͵puocat
urınā & ē cōuẽıẽs atrıtıōı neruorū
& dolorıbus matrıcıs .

.THYMVS.

Aſce.i.thymus. D.eſt plāta
nota oıbus & ē arbuſtū puū ī
q̃tıtate tára q̃ poſſūs accıpe ex rāu
lıs eıus & ıuoluere cırca eos cotū &
utı ͵p lıcınıo ad ıgnem accẽdẽdū &
b̃e folıa pua mıuta mſ̃ıum ſtrıcta
& oblōga.ı ſumıtatıbus eıus ſūt ca
pırella pua ſıcut formıce cırcūuolu
ta ıuıcẽ & tota plāta eıus ē breuıs
nō eleuat͛a terra mſ̃ıū & ē dura lı
gnoſa ſılr̃ & rāulı ſūt lıgnoſı & floſ
eıus ē purpureı colorıs & plurımū
q̃ ex ea naſcıt͛ē ı locıs petroſıs & aſ
pıs. G.virtus eıus prıa calefacıt
& deſıcat ı.ııı.gr̃.ſecūda ıncıdıt. &
tertıa ͵puocat urıam & mẽſtrua &
pellıt fetū & apıt opılatıōes uıſcer̃
& cōfr̃ excreatuı pectrıs ac pulcıs
D.uırtus eıus ē calefacta multū &
deſıcatā & ē cōuenıẽs ſtō ac pectorı
Quādo ſūıt͛ın potu cū ſale & aceto
laxat chım groſſū & fleuatıcū & q̃ū
amıſtrat͛decoctıo eıus cū melle con
fer̃ dıfıcultatı anelıtus ı q̃ oportet
bōıne erıgı & aſmatı & expellıt lō_
brıcos lōgos & ͵puocat urınā & q̃ū
cōfıcıt͛cum melle & fıt ıde lohoc ex
cludıt ſupfluıtates a pectore & q̃ū
fıt ẽpſm ex eo cū aceto reſoluıt apo
ſtẽıta fleuatıca dum ſūt noua & re
ſoluıt ſągıınē coagulatū & euellıt
emoroydas q; ſūt ı ano & uerucas

FIGURE 17.

ers, two totally anonymous books on botanical simples now missing, and the totally absent Serapion. It is possible that all of those books existed at one time and have since been lost or destroyed. However, it is also possible that Simon was attaching the names of earlier authorities to his own work, which was not an uncommon practice in his time.

Within Serapion's text there are plant names with a characteristically Spanish spelling, such as Xambar for Chambar, or Ouasima for Guasima. That would be the consequence of a method of translation used in Moorish Spain, where an Arabic text was often put into Spanish by either an Arab or a Jew, and then into Latin by a Spanish scholar. There is also evidence that some of the technical terms have been improperly translated from the original Arabic.

One historian of Arabic medicine, Lucien Leclerc, states that Serapion seems to have issued from a Hebrew manuscript rather than an Arabic one. At Paris he found an incomplete Hebrew manuscript, classed simply as a "Traité des Drogues," which lacked both beginning and end. It starts with the plant *Rubia tinctorum*, and ends with a kind of spurge that is termed camelea, but nowhere does the name of its originator appear. Leclerc states that it is a translation of the text of Serapion wherein are quoted Dioscorides' descriptions of plants and Galen's remarks on their properties, exactly as mentioned at the head of the *Liber de simplici medicina* by Serapion. There emerges the possibility that Simon Januensis may have bestowed the name of Serapion upon the work of an anonymous Jewish physician, so the mystery deepens.

FIGURE 18. Title page, Serapion, 1525 ed. Serapion was usually printed in combination with other herbals, such as this edition of 1525 by Jacob Myt of Lyons, which was certainly a bargain. Besides Serapion it contained works by Platearius, famous Magister of Salerno, and the Thesaurus Pauperum of Peter of Spain, who was also known as Pope John XXI when he was not advising on cheap home-remedies for the poor. (From *Practica Jo. Serapionis*. Lyon, Jacob Myt, 1525. Original size 5 5/16" wide × 8 1/2" high.)

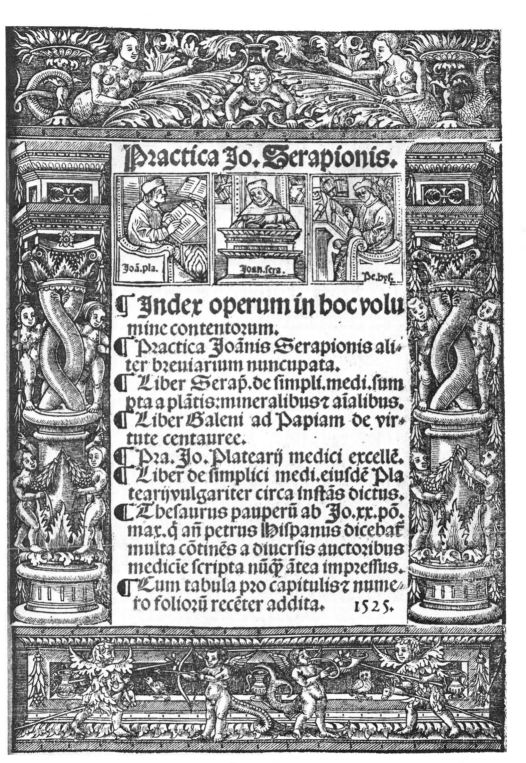

Practica Jo. Serapionis.

Joã.pla.

Joan.feps.

pe.hpſ.

❡ Index operum in hoc volu
mine contentorum.
❡ Practica Joānis Serapionis ali
ter breuiarium nuncupata.
❡ Liber Serap.de simpli.medi.sum
pta a plātis:mineralibus7 aialibus.
❡ Liber Galeni ad Papiam de vir
tute centauree.
❡ Pra. Jo. Platearij medici excellē.
❡ Liber de simplici medi.eiuſdē Pla
tearijvulgariter circa inſtās dictus.
❡ Thesaurus pauperū ab Jo.xx.pō.
max.q̃ añ petrus Ihiſpanus dicebat
multa cōtinēs a diuerſis auctoribus
medicie scripta nūcꝗ̃ ātea impreſſus.
❡ Cum tabula pro capitulis7 nume
ro foliorū recēter addita. 1525.

Figure 18.

No matter who wrote it, the book itself did much to spread the advanced medical knowledge of the Arabs throughout Europe. In addition to Greek and Arab sources, it quoted Persian and Indian ones as well. It outdid in popularity all other Arabic works, including that of the formidable Avicenna, whose work appeared in 21 editions before 1501. Serapion is cited some 976 times in the *Herbarius latinus, Der Gart,* and the *Hortus sanitatis,* three of the major early herbals, compared to a mere 533 mentions of Avicenna. Even as late as the 18th century he is quoted in Quincy's *Pharmacopeia officinalis, the London Dispensatory.* The case is similar to that of Mesue, whose work was used in the time of James I during the compilation of the London Pharmacopeia. But despite his popularity, only three editions of Serapion were printed in the incunabula period, which is yet another anomaly connected to his work.

BIBLIOGRAPHIC NOTES

Mesue, or Masāwaih al-Māradīnī. *De consolatione medicinarum, Grabadin, et Liber medicinarum particularum.*

Original manuscripts not extant.

1st edition: *De medicinis universalibus.* 1471 at Venice by Clemens Patavinus. In Latin.
1st illustrated edition: *Opera quae extant omnia.* 1561 at Venice by Vincentio Valgrisio.

Serapion or ibn Sārabiyūn. *Liber Serapionis aggregatus.*

Original manuscript not extant.

1st edition: 1473 at Milan by Antonius Zarotus of Parma. In Latin.

❧ 6 ❧

The *Circa Instans* of Matthaeus Platearius

HE *Circa instans* is a fundamental work of western science, but one that has been bedeviled by obscurity twice over. Its first period of neglect began when the larger printed herbals of the 16th century were favored over the *Circa*, with its modest dimensions. The second occurred when it began to be overlooked by bibliographers and historians of science and became unknown to all but a small group of specialists. This last fate is undeserved, for the *Circa* is the prototype of the modern pharmacopeia, the first attempt to establish nomenclatural standards, and the first effort by medieval physicians to create a work that did not echo the past. It made a point of providing information that was as accurate as possible for its era, and it shunned the superstition that pervaded so much of western culture at the time.

The book was conceived in response to problems that were pressing at the time and with which most physicians were unprepared to cope. These had to do with the basic substances used in medicine, the simples, so called because

45

they were the single, primary ingredients from which compounded prescriptions were made. There was much confusion also about some of the names found in medical writings that had been left over from ancient times. Many of these were either no longer understood or created a chaos that hampered communication. There was also the need to know which drugs were truly effective, and improved ways of administering them. Another problem was that of testing purity and quality. Because of restored and increased contact with the Asiatic world, many drugs of exotic origin had reappeared in the European market, where their now unfamiliar aspect opened the door to fraudulent practices. The *Circa*'s opening words announced its intentions: "About the present difficulty with the medicinal simples our treatise may be employed. . . ." Its aim was successfully achieved. Copies were circulated throughout Europe, where its value was instantly recognized and where it shaped the literature of botany and pharmacy for the next 300 years.

Although essentially a collective work of the School of Salerno, the leading medical center of the early Middle Ages, it is attributed by most medical historians to Matthaeus Platearius, one of the School's foremost teaching physicians. Within the text there are some references to cures that were identified with the Platearii, a family of medical practitioners who had already established a reputation at Salerno for their skill. The legendary Dame Trot or Trotula, famed as one of the first woman doctors, is said to have been the wife of one of the Platearii, but she may be an

FIGURE 19. Incipit *Circa instans,* 1497 ed. Although prototypes of illustrations had been created at Salerno in the 12th century to provide patterns for depicting medicinal plants, no printed edition of the Salernitan masterpiece, the *Circa instans,* was ever issued with pictures. This page shows the text of the *Circa*'s prologue and the chapter on Aloes in the rare first edition done at Venice in 1497. Its only decoration is to be found in the Renaissance-style initial letters. (From *Serapion liber aggregatus.* Venice, Bonetum Locatellum, 1497. Block of type 8" wide × 12" high.)

¶Platearius ve simplici medicina   186

℃Incipit liber ve simplici medicina secundū ↄplateariū. victus Circa instans.

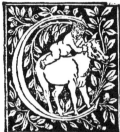

Irca instās ne/ go/ cium ve simplicib° medi/ cinie nostᵹ versaᵲ ↄpposi/ tū.Sipleᵹ āt medicina ē: que talis ē qualis a natu/ ra ↄvuciᵲ : vt gariofilus: nuᵹ muscata ⁊ silia:vel ᵹ licet aliquo sit mutata ar/ tificio:nó est aliᵹ medicie cōmixta: vt tamarindi:ᵹ abiectis ↄorticibus artifi/ cio ↄquassanᵲ:⁊ aloen ᵹ᳐ eᵹ berbe succo artificiose excocto efficiᵲ.℃Questio aūt nó ociosa ↄpponiᵲ .cur me/ dicine cōposite fuerit inuente:cum ois virtus que i cōpo/ sitis inest:in simplicib° repiaᵲ.Medicina aūt pᵹ morbi causam fertur extitisse inuēta.Dis aūt morbi cā fit aut eᵹ bumoᵹ abūdātia:aut eᵹ inanitóe:aut eᵹ fluᵹu:aut eᵹ vebilitate vtutum:aut eᵹ alteratóe qualitatū vel eᵹ solu tóe ↄtinuitatis.Inuemiᵲ aūt medicina simpleᵹ repletóis solutiua:⁊ inanitóis restauratiua:ↄstrictiua fluᵹ°:ↄforta tiua vebilitatis alteratióis imutatiua.solutióis ↄsolida/ tiua.℃Solutio.cōpositóis medicinaᵹ multipleᵹ cā eᵹ/ ᵲtit:s.morbi violétia.morboᵹ ↄrietas:membroᵹ ↄria vif positio:nobilitas mēbri : violentia medicinaᵹ.morbi.n. violétia:vt lepra appopla epilepsia:ᵹ simplicib° medicis aut viᵹ aut nuᵹ curanᵲ.Oportuit itaᵹᵹ adesse cōpositas ᵹt caᵹ virtute augmétata eᵹ simplicibus facilior fiat cu ratio egritudis violēte.Cótrarius morbis i eodē corpore ↄcurrétibus.vt febre leucoflegmātia eᵹ calo ⁊ frido cōposita extitit necessaria vt ᵹpetatib°ᵲᵹᵹs mor bis cótrarius valeat obuiare:vna.n.⁊ eadē medicia sim/ pleᵹ ᵲᵹᵹs qualitatibus affecta nó reperitur.Membris .n.ↄrarijs qualitatib°affectis existétib°:vt stó frido:cpe calo necessaria fuit medicia cōposita:vt ᵲᵹᵹs ᵹlitatib° mēbroᵹ ēt ↄtrarias qualitates possit alterare.Et mēbro etiā nobili:vtpote epate sclirosiᵹ patiēte necia fuit medi cia ↄposita:vt caso vissolo supflui fiat:⁊ stiptico ↄfortatio nobil'mēbri.Solū.n.casa nobile mēbᵹ exoluēdo vebili tat nisi stipticitate ↄfóteᵲ.Uioléta ēt mediᵲ:vtpote sca. elſa.⁊ silia simplᵲ vari nó vebét:nisi alie cōmiscanᵲ caᵹ violentiam alterátes.℃In tractatóc vniuscuiusᵹᵹ me/ dicine simplicᵢ cópᵲo reᵹ pē itendēda.ↄⁿr vtᵹ sit arbor an fruteᵹ.berba radiᵹ:an flos:an semen:an folium:an la pis:an succus:an aliᵹd alió. postmodū quot sunt ipſi'ᵐa neriᵲe:⁊ ᵹliter fiāt:⁊ i quo loco inueniaᵲ . ᵹ ēt maneries sit melior:ᵹliter ᵲᵹpseruari possunt:⁊ quas ᵲᵹtu.bēant: ⁊ qualᵲ ve bent eᵹhibi:⁊ pordinē alphabeti speᵹ tractatio cōpleaᵲ.

i	De aloe.	15 De allio.	29 De arnoglossa. 32 De assaro. 35 De anagalidos.
z	De ligno aloes.	16 De acoro.	30 De auena. 33 De ameos. 36 De apio cerfo.
3	De auro.	17 De amoniaco.	3i De abrotano. 34 De aaron.
4	De assa fetida.	18 De aniso.	
5	De argéto viuo.	19 De absinthio.	
6	De agno casto.	20 De anacardo.	
7	De alumine.	zi De amigdalis amaris.	
8	De apio.	zz De aristologia.	
9	De amido.	z3 De ambra.	
10	De antimonio.	z4 De arthemisia.	
ii	De acacia.	z5 De aceto.	
iz	De agarico.	z6 De alcanna.	
i3	De aneto.	z7 De auropigmento.	
14	De affodillo.	z8 De aspalto.	

℃De aloe.   I.

Aloes ca.⁊ sic. Aloes eᵹ succo berbe fit ᵹ ber ba suo noie aloe appellatur.bec āt berba nó solū i india ᵲperfia ⁊ grecia:veᵹ etiā i apulia repiᵲ.℃Aloes tria sūt gña:cicotrinū epaticū:caballinū.fit āt aloes ß mó.berba teriᵲ succus exprimiᵲ ad igné poniᵲ ᵹusᵹᵹ buliaᵲ.ᵹpostᵹᵹ bulierit ab igne remoueᵲ soli expóiᵲ ⁊ exiccaᵲ.Et vt ᵹda vicunt ᵹo supiᵒ est colligiᵲ ᵹo puriᵒest ⁊ cicotrinū vᵲ.ᵹo i medio ē minᵒpuᵹ ē ⁊ ↄepaticū appellaᵲ.ᵹo i fūdo ē feculē tū est ⁊ caball'.appellaᵲ.quoᵹ opio falsa ē.Tlos aūt vici mus:ᵹ viuerse sunt berbe nó in gñc:sᵹ i bonitate.Eᵹ gb° iste tres maneries aloes fiūt:sicut viuerse sunt vuc nó in gñc:sᵹ i bonitate.Eᵹ gb° vina fiunt vᵲia. ℃Optimū aūt aloes ē cicotrinū:⁊ viscerniᵲ eᵹ citrio colore aut subᵹufo: ⁊ ᵲpcipue cū frangiᵲ:cuius puluis apparet ᵹsi puluis croci eēt:⁊ eᵹ suba clara:⁊ maxime cū ᵲpminuta frāgiᵲ frusta:⁊ purā ⁊ subtilē ᵹ ᵹsi vesiccatā bᵹ subaᵹ.ᵹ leuiter frāgiᵲ:⁊ eᵹ eo ᵹ ᵹo ñ ē fetidū:nec valde amaᵹ:⁊ ᵹnᵹᵹ gūmosū:ᵹñ/ ᵹᵹ frāgibile.℃Epaticū colori epis assimilaᵲ.bᵹ āt coloᵲᵲ epaᵲ:fed fubnigᵹ:⁊ binc inde foramina babet vt ora ve/ narum:obscuram babet substantiam:⁊ non claram:⁊ alia signa predictis similia que omnia babet remissiora:⁊ ma xime colorem.℃Caballiuᵹ vero nigrum:⁊ obscurum ē ⁊ feculentam babet substantiam:amarissimū:⁊ borribi lem pretendit odorem:qᵲ valde fetidum est.Sophistica tur autem caballinum:vt cicotrinu seu epaticū videaᵲ Qᵲ autem ve sophisticatione buius ⁊ aliarum specierᵹ rogatu sociorum scripsimus:ad sophisticationes vitādas ⁊ fraudulentias conficientium ⁊ vendentiuᵹ fecimus:nó vt ab aliquo committatur sophisticatio : sed vt fraudu lenta veuiretur veceptio.virtus enim sese viligit:⁊ asper naᵲ contraria:nec potest vitari vitium nisi cognitum. ℃Sophisticatur autem aloe boc modo:buliat acetum: ⁊ addito puluere croci orietalis:⁊ puluere modico nucis muscate:vel alterius speciei odorifere:Caballinum auté aloen per frusta parua viuisum simul cum filis ligetur:⁊ in accto bulienti imittatur:⁊ subito cleuetur exiccari mo dicuᵹ vimittaᵲ:⁊ sic vecies aut amplius fiat ita ᵹᵹ coloᵹ ⁊ odoᵹ immutentur.ita ᵹᵹ videatur esse epaticum:seu cico/ trinum:⁊ exiccari modicuᵹ permittatur:⁊ vifficile cogno scitur ᵹo non sic:viscernitur tamen:qᵲ cum frangitur ⁊ vi gitis ↄfricatur statim fetidissimum sentiᵲ:ᵹo in epati co seu cicotrio nó ē.℃Et nota ᵹo vó ᵹo nā ē aromᵲ: quāto plus ē aromaticū tāto meli°:eᵹᵲ oē ᵹo nā sua est amaᵹ ᵹnto plus ē amaᵹ excepto aloc:tāto meli°:⁊ oē ᵹo nālᵲ ē fetidū:ᵹᵹto fetidᵒ:tāto meli°:excepto aloc:⁊ oē ᵹo oᵹ bēre aliᵹd saporᵲ:ᵹnto i sapoᵲe lio iteſiᵒ ē tāto meliᵒ excepto aloen:ᵹo cū sit naturaliter amarum quanto mi nus:amarum tanto laudabilius.

℃Aloen vo bᵹ purgare co.⁊ ſła ⁊ mūdificat meliaᵹ.bᵹ ēt ᵲrutē ↄfortatú mēbᵲ neruosa.vñ valᵹ ᵲᵹ supfluitatē frido rū bu.i stó ↄtétoᵲ:ipᵹ āt stóᵹ ↄfortat:caput a volore ele uat:ᵹ eᵹ amabamiasi.fit.i.cᵹ fuositate stói.visū clāificat. opilós splēis ⁊ epis apiᵲ:méstrua ᵲuocat:supfluitate cē pudēda:si sint eᵹ frida cā extergit:scabie ēt curat.cōᵲᵒ vif coloᵲatū reddit coloratū:si fuerit viscoloratū eᵹ ᵲcedēti egritudie:valet ēt ᵹ alopiciā.i. casuᵹ capilloᵹ.℃Si bu flatic° ⁊ meliᵲᵒ abūdauerint i stóᵲᵹ pi vigóneᵹ vēᵲ.ᵹ.y. aloes cū.ᵹ.i.mastici stóᵹ mūdificat:⁊ eudē vbilitatū ⁊ ifri datū ↄfortat.āt idē:ᵹnuᵹ aloes cū melle eᵹhibitū valeᵲ: si propter abbominationem aliter accipi non potest:stó macbium mundificat:⁊ vigestionem procurat:⁊ nota ᵹᵹ aloes ⁊ mastiᵹ vebent ↄteri:⁊ cū ᵹino albo vecoᵹ:⁊ vari.

FIGURE 19.

apocryphal figure representing all the Salernitan women connected with medicine. Elsewhere in the text is a statement in the first person referring to a painful discharge of urine, which says that "By this remedy I, Platearius, was freed." The passage occurs in his discussion of the plant called strucium (our Soapwort, Bouncing Bet, or *Saponaria officinalis*). Since Matthaeus was the leading member of the Platearii at the time the *Circa* was written, about 1140–50, and was also the author of a very popular commentary on the *Antidotarium* of Nicolaus of Salerno, it is reasonable to suppose that he was entrusted with the task of setting down the collective opinions of the Salernitan school.

The first printed edition of the *Circa instans* contained 273 "chapters," though they are better termed items, for some of them are only a line or two in length. Most of the discussions are on botanically derived drugs. Some 229 plants are named, which gives it importance for our knowledge of 12th-century botany. The manuscript versions are usually somewhat shorter, hovering around 250 to 260 chapters, so it is presumed that the extra headings found in the printed *Circa* are not part of the original text.

Although the *Circa* had been of prime importance until the beginning of the 15th century, its appeal waned with the appearance of the comprehensive printed herbals. They cited it frequently, and may thus have delayed a separate printing of it. When it did reach print it was bound with other works, notably the *Liber aggregatus* of Serapion the Younger. The early bibliographers of botany, Haller and Seguier, listed the *Circa*, but Pritzel's *Thesaurus literaturae botanicae*, a botanist's Bible if there ever was one, neglects it entirely. The only clue to its existence in Pritzel comes under Platearius, and consists of a reference to Ernst Meyer's *Geschichte der Botanik* wherein Platearius is discussed. Thus poor Platearius was buried almost without a trace.

Neglect of the *Circa* continued into the present century. Two editions of *Incunabula in American Libraries* fail to list

Platearius separately, subordinating him instead under Serapion. Even the estimable *Incunabula Scientifica et Medica* of Arnold Klebs does little to remedy the situation. It does list the *Circa instans* and Platearius, but devotes its major heading to Serapion's *Liber aggregatus,* with which the *Circa* was printed. Bibliographies sometimes conceal a book as much as reveal it. Once a book is discovered, however, it is yet another matter to locate a copy. Manuscripts of the *Circa* are very rare, and only fourteen printed copies are in the U.S. Even if found, a manuscript would be hard to decipher since many such texts are in the form of scribal symbols and contractions, which were in turn carried over into early printed books. One is reminded of the buggy-whip that adorned many of the first automobiles.

Fortunately for the *Circa* and Platearius, the history of science has been developing as a field for some time now, and there the *Circa* is given its just due. Ernst Meyer placed it on a par with Pliny and Dioscorides. Edward Sanford Burgess termed it the center of medieval botany, and the source for the next three centuries of growth in that field. George Sarton saw it as a great improvement over Dioscorides and other herbal writings, and both Lynn Thorndike and Claus Nissen spoke of it with respect.

Of course modern science has long since outgrown the *Circa,* just as Newton surpassed Euclid, and Einstein overshadowed Newton, but each built on work that had gone before, and gladly acknowledged their debt. The *Circa* may not be consulted nowadays in the prescription room of your corner drugstore, nor in pharmaceutical laboratories, but it was a major instrument in making those places possible.

BIBLIOGRAPHIC NOTES

Original manuscript no longer extant, but estimated c. 1130–50. Oldest extant versions are now in the NYBG Library: Manuscript A dates from c.1190 (formerly known as Ms. Starkenstein A).

Manuscript B dates from c. 1200 to c. 1225 (formerly known as
Ms. Starkenstein B).

Ms. M 1302, Codex Salernitanus, once in the University Library at
Wroclaw, Poland, which included the *Circa instans* in its con-
tents and was estimated to date from c. 1180, perished during
World War II.

A manuscript in the National Library in Vienna, Ms. 2461, contains *Circa instans* on leaves 163r–200v. Its script is in a style
dating from no later than 1250, which implies that it has mid-
13th-century characteristics and thus is of a later date than either of NYBG's manuscripts.

1st edition: 1497 at Venice by Bonetum Locatellum for Octaviani
Scoti. Bound with Serapion's *Liber aggregatus*.

A Ferrarese edition of 1488 is often cited as *editio princeps*, particularly in books from before 1940. Klebs and Goff both ignore it,
and it should be considered a "ghost," a phantom edition
created by a bibliographer's error.

❧ 7 ❧

The *Physica* of Hildegarde of Bingen

OUGHLY contemporary with the *Circa instans* is the *Physica* of Hildegarde of Bingen. Her work is notable for several reasons. It is the first book in which a woman discusses plants and trees in relation to their medicinal properties. It is the earliest book on natural history to be done in Germany, and is, in essence, the foundation of botanical study there. It influenced the 16th-century works of Brunfels, Fuchs, and Bock, the so-called "German fathers of botany," but the fact is that German botany is more indebted to a "mother."

It is all the more remarkable that Hildegarde wrote a book so strongly concerned with science, for all of her other works are of a mystical and theological nature. Born in 1099 in the little German town of Böckelheim on the River Nahe, near Mainz, she was the daughter of a knight. For some reason, possibly for economy, protection, or recognition of exceptional talent, she was placed in the Benedictine convent at Disibodenberg at the age of eight. There she was under the care of the Abbess Jutta, who saw to her education. Hildegarde became her successor as Abbess in 1136.

From early childhood Hildegarde was subject to visions, which became ever more frequent, intense, and vivid as she attained maturity. That fact was concealed to a considerable extent until she reached the age of 42, when she began to write about them. Once her visions became known throughout the religious community they evoked great interest, and St. Bernard of Clairvaux, who met her at Bingen while preaching the Second Crusade, became convinced that she was a true prophetess of God. Recommendation from that quarter led to further recognition by the dignitaries of the Church, including Pope Eugenius III.

In 1148, perhaps to retreat somewhat from her newfound celebrity, Hildegarde took eighteen of her nuns from Bingen and with them established a new convent at Rupertsberg where she remained as Abbess until her death in 1179. In addition to her gifts as a mystic, Hildegarde had quite a reputation for her learning. She was in correspondence with Popes, Emperors, and leading theologians, one of whom, Guibert of Gembloux, submitted questions on dogma to Hildegarde for her opinion. Despite her sheltered life in the convent, Hildegarde made a number of journeys out into the world and exercised considerable influence on the religious thought of her age. Her influence was greater than her provincial origin and setting would seem to have permitted.

The *Physica*, or Natural Science, which brought her renown beyond the realm of religious mysticism, is more than a book of natural history, for it has had a decided emphasis on the practice of medicine. At first glance this may seem a strange work for a cloistered nun, but it is, in fact, an outgrowth of her duties in the convent. In the 12th century, and most particularly north of the Alps, which was far from Salerno, the practice of medicine was still largely in the hands

COSMAS.   DAMIANVS.

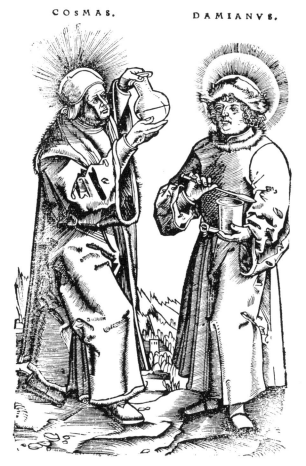

FIGURE 20. Cosmas and Damian. Patron saints of medicine, Cosmas and Damian were brothers skilled in that art, which they practiced free of charge for all who needed their help. They were beheaded at the command of the proconsul Lisias after the executioners had tried a variety of other techniques without success. Posthumously they were declared to be saints, and a series of miracles were ascribed to them. Not the least of those was the invention of the transplant; they substituted the leg of a dead Moor for a cancerous one belonging to a devotee of theirs. (From Hildegarde's *Physica*. *Strassburg, J. Schott*, 1533. Original size 5″ wide × 8 ¹/₈″ high.)

T Y P V s Infirmitatum & Paſſionum accidens
tium corpori humano ab intra.

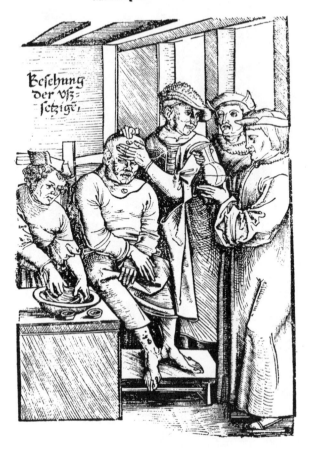

FIGURE 21. Physicians consulting. Another medically pertinent block inserted in Schott's edition of
the *Physica* was this consultation of physicians
around their client. They may be deciding to cut the
stone of folly (thought to be in the forehead, where
it caused stupidity and mental disorder), or they
may be simply making up their minds as to whether
or not he should be bled, and where. Since a basin
is already present the patient will probably soon feel
the lancet. (From Hildegarde's *Physica*. Strassburg,
J. Schott, 1533. Original size 5″ wide × 8 5/16″ high.)

T Y P V s morborum & plagarum acciden=
tium ab extra corpori humano.

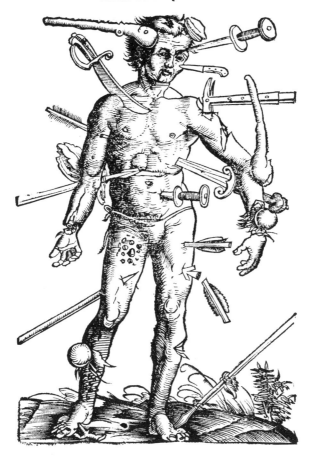

FIGURE 22. Wound Man. This battered and be-
leagured individual, looking rather like a casualty of
modern inner-city living, is actually a visual table of
contents that had seen earlier use in works on
surgery. Since no illustrations had ever been done
for Hildegarde's *Physica,* the publisher, Johann
Schott, was forced to use whatever blocks he had on
hand that might have any connection with medicine. (From Hildegarde's *Physica.* Strassburg,
J. Schott, 1533. Original size 5″ wide × 8 ⁵/₁₆″ high.)

of the clergy. Not only were monks and nuns treated in the abbeys and convents of the religious orders, but also those who worked on their lands, villagers of the nearby parishes, and wayfarers, whom the Christian faith exhorted its faithful to treat with charity and mercy.

It is understandable, then, why Hildegarde absorbed so much medical knowledge. Her *Physica,* in addition to displaying the state of knowledge then existing about the natural world, gives us a reliable picture of how medicine was practiced by the clergy. She included recipes handed down by generations of her predecessors, her own observations of diseases and cures, and various folk-remedies. In the course of gathering such information she frequently came upon plant names that were not translatable into Latin. Faced with that difficulty the very practical Hildegarde simply kept the original and, thanks to her, we have the first recorded use of such names as Hymelsluszel (Heaven's keys) for the primrose (*Primula vulgaris*), Storcksnabel and Cranchsnabel for two species of geraniums, and Hufflatich for Tussilago (coltsfoot). There are numerous others of interest to those concerned with the development of the German language, and Hildegarde's work deserves more study than it has received in the past. The great medical historian and bibliographer, Ludwig Choulant, assigned her book greater importance than many more learned works on the basis of what it revealed about folk-medicine in her time.

One remedy that Hildegarde suggests for women having difficulty in labor will strike most readers as a bit impractical and nonsensical: she recommends placing a lion's heart on the navel of the pregnant woman, but only for a brief space of time. This was supposed to ease the birth. Where anyone was apt to come upon a lion in Bavaria in Hildegarde's day she does not say, nor does she suggest a way of getting the creature to relinquish such a necessary organ.

Other quotes reveal more sensibility, especially when

they are connected to matters within Hildegarde's own experience. They are in general, however, strongly colored by the beliefs of her day, which were built on dim memories and notions from the past, many of them akin to those of Apuleius. Peas, for instance, were considered inferior to beans as a food, and more apt to cause internal troubles. Hempseed was thought to be a relief for headaches, nutmeg purified the senses and lessened evil humours, and rose leaves when placed upon the eyes would remove dirt and foreign matter, clarifying the sight. Such things had been said for a thousand years before, and they would continue to be said until the 19th century. It is not their efficacy that is in question, nor should we censure Hildegarde for repeating them; what does matter is that she gives us an unretouched view into the beliefs and practices of medieval man. In our part of the world medieval man has only just gone around the corner, one heel still visible, while elsewhere, in Asia and Africa, he is very much with us. We can perhaps understand ourselves better by knowing more about him, and one of Hildegarde's virtues is that she makes that possible. Another is that she undertook a task of encyclopedic scope at least a century before other more famous writers, such as Vincent of Beauvais and Bartholomaeus Anglicus, wrote their works. She also knew the practical steps in baking a loaf of bread, unlike Bartholomew, who skimmed over the details of the process in this fashion: "and at last after many travailes, man's lyfe is fedde and sustained therewith."

BIBLIOGRAPHIC NOTES

Original manuscript not extant. Estimated time of composition c. 1150.
Date and location of earliest manuscript unavailable at present time.

1st edition: 1533 at Strassburg by Johann Schott. It is also the first illustrated edition, but the three woodcuts that accompany it were used earlier for works on surgery and medicine. They have no real relation to Hildegarde's text, and were used simply because the publisher wanted to dress up the book with pictures from his stock.

ᵔ᷉ 8 ᷆ᵕ

Bartholomaeus Anglicus:
De Proprietatibus Rerum

 A R T H O L O M E W was an Englishman, as the epithet Anglicus implies, but he does not seem to have taken his nationality as seriously as did those who named him, for much of his schooling took place in Paris, where he elected to stay and teach. After that he resided in Magdeburg, Saxony. There is a possibility that he was influenced by Robert Grosseteste in an early period of study at Oxford. His interest in natural science offers some support for that supposition, but it is actually more likely that Albertus Magnus was his mentor.

A member of the Minorite Order, he was also a professor of theology at Paris until the year 1230, when the General of the Friars' Minor (Franciscans) in Saxony requested that Bartholomew and one other monk be sent to him. What prompted the need is lost to history, as is so much else of Bartholomew's life, but it must have been considered necessary by his superior, the Provincial of France, for he went to Magdeburg and remained there for the next 45 years, very likely the remainder of his life. That he wrote *De proprieta-*

tibus rerum (Of the Properties of Things) is the only other certainty that can be stated in connection with him, but when and where he wrote it is unknown.

Bartholomew's book was written in Latin sometime before 1283, for by then it was already known in Italy. Subsequently it was translated into French, English, Dutch, and Spanish, and mention is made of a version in Bavarian. About 25 editions of *De proprietatibus rerum* were printed before the end of the incunabula period, a sure sign of the popularity it had evoked from the very beginning. The first of those printed editions is held by Sarton to be the one done at Basle by Berthold Ruppel. It bears no date but is said to have been printed about 1470–72. Another edition, which lacks place, date, and printer, is held by some bibliographers to have been printed at Cologne in 1470–71 by William Caxton.

Bartholomew's encyclopedia (for that is the only appropriate term for it) met with instant approval at the universities which were then springing up throughout Europe. It seems to have filled a need not fully met by earlier works, such as those of Pliny and Isidore of Seville. Rivals to it were the great *Natura rerum* of Thomas de Cantimpré and the *Speculum majus tripartitum* of Vincent of Beauvias, but Bartholomew seems to have been most successful. The *Natura rerum* was never printed, and Vincent's *Speculum* was too overwhelming in length to hold any but the most avid and persistent readers. At Paris, however, Bartholomew's manuscript was in brisk enough demand to be rented to scholars

FIGURE 23. Title page of *De proprietatibus rerum* (detail). Bartholomaeus Anglicus created the most famous of medieval encyclopedias when he wrote *De proprietatibus rerum* (Of the Properties of Things). This detail from the title page of a Spanish edition (Toledo, 1529) gives an idea of its scope and concerns. Religion, natural history, geography, medicine, astronomy, and household affairs form only part of its contents. (From *Libro de proprietatibus rerum en romance*. Toledo, Gaspar de Avila for Joan Thomas Fabio, 1529. Original size of detail 6 3/4" wide × 7" high.)

Libro de proprietatibus rerum en romance.

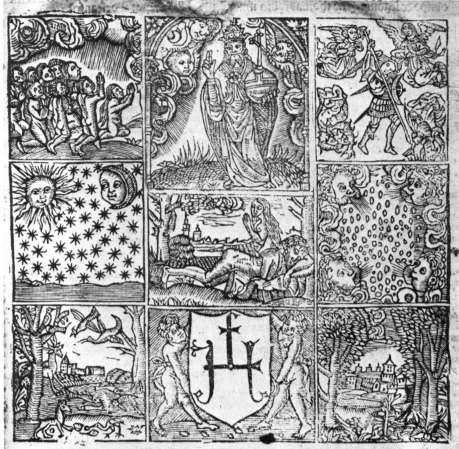

Hystoria natural: do se tratã las ppiedades d̃ todas las cosas
Es obra catholica τ muy puechosa: que cõtiene mucha dotrina de theologia: hablãdo
de dios: τ mucha filosofia moral τ natural hablando de sus criaturas. Va acopañada de
grãdes secretos de astrologia: medicina: cirugia: geometria: musica τ cosmografia. Cõ
otras sciencias en. xx. libros siguientes.

Libro. j. de dios τ su esencia.
El. ij. dlos ãgeles buenos τ malos
El. iij. del anima.
El. iiij. dlos huõres y elemẽtos.
El. v. del hõbre y sus partes
El. vj. delas hedades
El. vij. delas enfermades
El. viij. d̃l cielo y mũdo: τ plãetas

El nouene d̃l tiempo.
El. x. dela materia τ forma.
El. xj. del ayre: τ sus impresiones
El. xij. delas aues.
El. xiij. delas aguas
El. xiiij. dela tierra τ mõtañas
El. xv. delas prouincias d̃l mũdo
El. xvj. delas piedras τ metales.

El. xvij. dlos arbõles plãtas: τ yruas
El. xviij. delos animales.
El diez τ nueue delos colores: olo
res: sabores: licores: τ dlos hueuos
El. xx. τ vltimo delos numeros: τ
delas medidas τ pesos τ instru/
mentos y sones.

Lo qual todo por sus capitulos largamẽte se vera por la tabla.

FIGURE 23.

at regulated rates, well before the modern lending library had ever been conceived.

Bartholomew patterned his book on the *Etymologiarum libri duo* of the learned ecclesiastic, Isidore of Seville, which had been written between A.D. 622 and 633. Bartholomew reduced the number of parts, then called books, from the 20 found in Isidore to 19, and rearranged the order of topics. This does not mean that he plagiarized Isidore, nor for that matter any other author, but that his compilation adhered to an accepted form and was built upon what was then considered to be accurately stated knowledge. His own observations, however, permeate *De proprietatibus rerum* and give the work its unique flavor.

The 19 sections of Bartholomew's book follow this order: (1) God; (2) Angels and Demons; (3) Of the Soul and Reason; (4) Of the Body's Essences; (5) The Human Body and Each of its Parts; (6) The Ages of Man (Family Life and Household Economy); (7) Of Infirmities and Medicines; (8) Of the World and the Heavenly Bodies (Cosmology and Astrology); (9) Of Time and the Divisions of Time; (10) The Material, Form, and Properties of the Elements; (11) Of the Air and its Natural Phenomena (Meteorology); (12) Of Winged Creatures; (13) Of Waters and Fish; (14) Of the Earth and its Features; (15) Of its Provinces (Political and Economic Geography); (16) Mineralogy; (17) On Plants and Trees (A Herbal); (18) Of Animals; (19) On Non-Essential Characteristics (i.e., Colors, Tastes, Odors, etc.), and a Miscellany on Food, Drink, Eggs, Weights and Measures, Music, and Musical Instruments. In some respects Bartholomew's work resembles the modern encyclopedia, especially in its attempt to treat every possible subject, while in its final part it is more reminiscent of some dictionaries or almanacs that append a mixture of useful information to the main contents.

The order of the *Proprietatibus rerum* is founded on a medieval logic of progression. God, as the supreme creator and prime moving force, occupies the first position, and is immediately followed by the next most important factors to affect the life of man, the forces of good and evil. Since the spiritual salvation of man takes precedence over his physical welfare, his soul and his mind are discussed prior to the workings of his body, his family relationships, and his health. Last in the hierarchy is the world of nature in all its aspects from astronomy to animals. The purpose of this section is to provide man with exemplifications of good and bad conduct, to illustrate for him the precepts of Christianity.

Since the greatest importance was assigned to theological and teleological matters, it became fairly simple to disregard the accuracy of data and to consider observation of phenomena as an occupation fit for the lower orders of craftsmen. Hence we find Bartholomew with no clear idea of the locations of Egypt or India, the latter being a vague term which medieval men used to refer to the vast territory that stretched beyond Arabia. Bartholomew's own eyes would have told him that bees do not carry small stones to weight them against the wind, and that crabs do not employ stones to keep oyster shells propped open while they dine on the contents. It was as obvious then as now that the legs of a fox are not shorter on the right side, and that swiftly moving currents are not the cause of oars becoming disjointed in appearance when dipped under water. Yet we cannot blame him for being a man of his times. After all, we can hardly boast of our perfected wisdom when we skip from 12 to 14 in numbering a building's floors, or run horoscope columns in our daily papers.

The section of *De proprietatibus rerum* that most concerns this present work is Book 17, which discusses trees and plants. Most of its material is drawn from Isidore, Dioscorides, Pliny, and Platearius, who are repeatedly cited as Bartholomew's authorities, although occasional references are made to Avicenna, Macer, Hippocrates, and the Bible.

The treatise opens with a general discussion of the nature and properties of trees, in which he says that the life and virtues present in trees and plants are hidden and not made manifest as they are with animals. "Trees move not by voluntary motion, as animals do, nor are they affected by appetite, liking, or sadness. There is vegetative life in plants . . . but they lack the sensitivity of a soul. . . ." This is clearly a reference to Aristotle's theory that ranked the various forms of life in descending order from man to animal to plant, and since Bartholomew was a disciple of the Greek philosopher it was natural for him to voice the idea.

Following the generalized prologue of Book 17 is a full-fledged herbal that mentions some 144 species. These are arrayed in loose alphabetical order, as was common then. For instance, Aloes comes before Absinthium, and Gramine before Galbanum, so that the alphabetizing stops after the initial letter. Since indices and pagination were often lacking, it was no simple matter to locate a specific passage in any of the medieval manuscripts, nor in the early printed works, so even rough alphabetization helped.

Bartholomew begins his herbal proper with Amigdalus (almond), and proceeds through Zuchara (sugar cane). The origins and meanings of the plant names are from the *Etymologiarum libri duo* of Isidore, but the bulk of their medicinal uses are from Dioscorides, the *Circa instans* of Platearius, or Pliny. Under Mandragora, in John of Trevisa's translation, we find this prescription: "The rind thereof medled with wine . . . gene to them to drink that shall be cut in their body for they should slepe and not fele the sore knitting." Such anesthesia had been known and used since classical times, patients often preferring its known danger (of causing death instead of sleep) to the pain that would have to be endured without it. Elsewhere he speaks of the rose, "Among all floures of the worlde the floure of the rose is cheyf and beereth ye pryse. And by cause of vertues and swete smelle and savour. For by fayrnesse they fede the syghte, and playseth the smelle by odour, the touche be soft handlynge. And wythstondeth and socouryth by vertue ayenst many syknesses and evylles." Despite the lapse of favor for the rose in modern medicine, Bartholomew's contemporaries and many generations after agreed with him. Perhaps the soothing qualities of the rose had a psychological effect that more pragmatic physicians chose to ignore.

But whatever the verdict concerning Bartholomew's medicaments we can be thankful that his division of time never gained the popularity that his encyclopedia did. Time, in Bartholomew's day, was anything but an exact science. The length of the hours was regulated by the length of daylight. Basse prime was at break of day and vespers at twilight (as the word implies), and what came between was roughly divided into such elastic segments as terce, sext, none—the third, sixth, and ninth hours after sunrise—but none of these hours were necessarily equal to our 60-minute hour. Bartholomew's system started out in an orderly fashion with a 24-hour day, but then it proposed to split each hour into 4 points of 10 moments each. Still worse, each moment was divided into 12 ounces, and each ounce was fragmented into 47 atoms. Later ages have been grateful to Bartholomew for the pleasure of learning his encyclopedia brought to them, and they have also been grateful to his contemporaries for letting his time-keeping method die an unmourned death.

BIBLIOGRAPHIC NOTES

Original manuscript not extant. Estimated time of composition between 1248 and 1260.

Earliest manuscript probably Ms. 1512 in Ashmolean Library at Oxford, which is dated 1296.

1st edition: not dated, but between 1470 and 1472 at Basle by Berthold Ruppel.

1st illustrated edition: 1482 at Lyons by Matthias Huss.

◄§ 9 §►

The *Opus Ruralium Commodorum* of Pietro Crescenzi

H E first major work on agriculture since the days of the Roman Empire was Crescenzi's *Opus ruralium commodorum,* or *The Advantages of Country-living.* Much of it, in fact, was culled from the writings of those old Roman authors who are termed the Scriptores Rei Rusticae: Cato, Columella, Varro, and Palladius. The traditions of agriculture embodied in their books were still in evidence in Crescenzi's time, as they are even to this day in the vineyards around Vesuvius.

Although there was little that was new or original in Crescenzi's work, it proved to be a popular one from the moment of its inception, and endured as an authority right down to the 18th century. Its first appearance in manuscript was c.1306, when Crescenzi had completed it. Some 132 manuscript copies with various dates are still in existence today, so the total number circulating up to the time of printing must have been very high. The book was printed in 1471, and was shortly followed by 16 other editions in the incunabula period, plus another 36 during the 1500s. All in all the *Opus ruralium commodorum* was an unqualified success, and the reasons are fairly plain to see when we consider the needs of a world that had to rely almost entirely on its local produce, horse-power, and ingenuity.

The contents of Crescenzi's book provided anyone who worked on the land with a well-organized manual of procedure. The *Opus ruralium commodorum* is divided into twelve sections, each of which addresses itself to a specific agricultural topic. Book I discusses the best location and arrangement of a manor, villa, or farm, and touches on every necessary point from proper water supply to the duties of the head of the household. Book II provides the farmer with the botanical background needed to raise every kind of crop. Book III tells how to build a granary and a threshing floor, and how to cultivate cereal, forage, and food crops. Book IV is on vines, wine-making, the means of preserving both fresh and dried grapes. Books V and VI are on arboriculture and horticulture, respectively. Book VII is on meadows and woods, while Book VIII, which contains a quantity of original material, is on gardens, and is very much the model for gardening books of the 16th and 17th centuries. Book IX concerns animal husbandry and bee-keeping (honey was then the major source for sweeteners). Book X is about hunting and fishing. Book XI offers a general summary of the work, and Book XII is a calendar of duties and tasks to be performed month by month.

Crescenzi's Books V and VI may be termed more properly a herbal. While the products of both orchard and kitchen-garden are spoken of in its pages, the greater emphasis is placed on medicaments made from fruits and herbs. In Crescenzi's day a country establishment of any size had to be as nearly self-reliant as possible. If medicines were needed for either men or animals there was little opportunity to get them from the corner drugstore. Instead they had to be raised, harvested, and preserved for use. Foresight was required if the farm was to prosper, and the

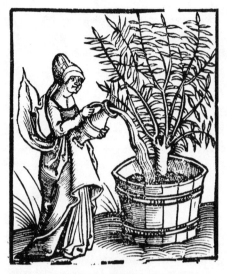

FIGURE 24. Rosemary. This herb was thought to thrive best in those households where the woman ruled. The lady so assiduously watering this splendid specimen seems to be taking no chances of losing command. Used today largely for flavoring lamb, rosemary was once a funeral herb, strewn for remembrance, and also was a moth preventative. It was believed to restore appetite, relieve gout, whiten the face, and preserve wine. (From *Von dem Nutzen der Dinge*. Strassburg, J. Schott, 1518. Original size 2 3/4" wide × 3 11/16" high.)

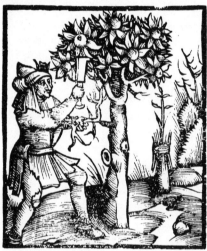

FIGURE 25. Pomegranate. The "apples of Africa," being harvested here with a medieval version of the machete, grew well enough in Crescenzi's Italy but were hardly dependable as an orchard crop for those reading the German translation. Even today the same kind of climatic oversight occurs in many horticultural works that make sense for the country in which they originated, but are not adapted to suit other climes. (From *Von dem Nutzen der Dinge*. Strassburg, J. Schott, 1518. Original size 2 3/4" wide × 3 11/16" high.)

manager of such a place had to be a Jack-of-all-trades. The *Opus ruralium commodorum* was a practical handbook for organizing the manifold chores about a farm, and a trouble-shooting guide whenever things went wrong.

Most of the medicinal information in Crescenzi is taken from the *Circa instans* of Platearius, which had already been

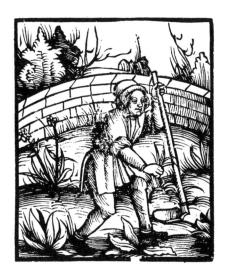

FIGURE 26. Borage. The herb being cultivated here (albeit with a hoe that seems capable of as much damage as the weeds it is supposed to eliminate) was once a staple item in herbal medicine. The leaves and flowers put into wine brought courage and merriment to the hearts of men, so it was said. If true, the 20th century could use as much of it as the 14th or the 1st, when Crescenzi and Dioscorides put it to that use. (From *Von dem Nutzen der Dinge.* Strassburg, J. Schott, 1518. Original size 2 ³/₄" wide × 3 ¹¹/₁₆" high.)

the standard authority for a century and a half by the time the *Opus ruralium commodorum* was written. The women of Salerno are cited by Crescenzi on several occasions, as are Pliny, Dioscorides, Galen, Avicenna, and Albertus Magnus. Platearius is not mentioned by name in the medicinal section although passages from his book are paraphrased throughout. Crescenzi regarded himself not as a creative writer tainted by plagiarism, but as a compiler, like Pliny, who was performing a labor of love that would benefit others far more than himself. Whatever the economics of publishing in those times, it is not likely that any author, including Crescenzi's contemporary, Dante, ever grew rich from royalties.

Throughout Crescenzi's early life he had developed a great interest in nature, and while a student at the University of Bologna, his native city, he studied natural science, medicine, and logic. Undoubtedly it was there that be became familiar with the *Circa instans.* Born around 1230 to 1233, he grew up in a time when the war between the Guelphs and the Ghibellines was reaching its climax. Bologna, at that time, was a Guelph (pro-Papal) stronghold, but the power struggle then going on sometimes gave the Ghibelline forces (pro-Emperor) the advantage. A great deal of Crescenzi's time was necessarily spent in less troubled areas, but daily living must still have been hazardous, for he practiced law and adjudicated cases in many of the towns of Italy.

Much of his legal work was done in the north of Italy. The Ghibelline faction was much stronger in the south around Naples and Sicily, where the Hohenstaufen dynasty held sway. The name Ghibelline, despite its Italianate sound, is simply a corruption of Waiblingen, which was a possession of Frederick II. Somehow Crescenzi escaped harm despite the violence of his times and retired in 1299 to his Villa d'Olmo (the Elms) at Urbizzano, some ten miles outside Bologna.

There he spent the remainder of his life doing what he had loved as a youth, tending to country affairs and the management of his estate, and writing a book on the subject. Sometime about 1306 he completed the work and released it to the world. It became so popular that it lasted more than 300 years. Composed in Latin, it was translated first into Italian, then French (some say he was acquainted with Provence), German, and finally Polish. Three chapters from his book on gardening were translated into English as late as 1924 by Sir Frank Crisp, so one cannot be entirely sure that the career of the *Opus ruralium commodorum* has come to a complete stop. For those who would like to get a sense of medieval life Crescenzi offers a satisfying dose of it, and if the reader is fortunate enough to come across the illustrated edition of 1495 he is certain to be delighted by the woodcuts, which breathe the charm of an earlier age. There peacocks strut within the garden of a crenellated castle, and coopers are binding the staves of huge wine casks. They are idyllic, calm, evocative of the peace that prevailed when Crescenzi dedicated his book to Charles II of Anjou. But,

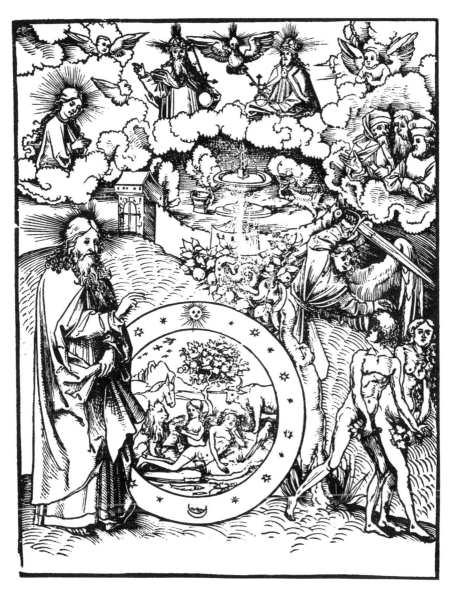

FIGURE 27. Creation and Expulsion of Man. In 1518 Johann Schott published *Von dem Nutzen der Dinge,* a German translation of Pietro Crescenzi's *Opus ruralium commodorum* (The Advantages of Country Living). In the more leisurely fashion of an earlier day, the illustrator began at the very beginning of agriculture with the expulsion of Adam and Eve from Eden. The first book of Crescenzi's work is just as basic, for it treats of the location of a farm and everything necessary to its proper management. (From *Von dem Nutzen der Dinge.* Strassburg, J. Schott, 1518. Original size 6 $^9/_{16}''$ wide × 8 $^9/_{16}''$ high.)

just as in the modern world, war broke out again and stayed for the remainder of Crescenzi's lifetime. Happily it did not prevent the Villa d'Olmo from passing quietly to his son in 1321 when, his long life over, the will of Pietro Crescenzi was probated.

BIBLIOGRAPHIC NOTES

Manuscript copies: over 130 known to exist as late as 1940. Location of oldest copy not known at this writing.

1st edition: 1471 at Augsburg by [Johann Schussler].

1st illustrated edition: between 1490 and 1495 at Speyer by Peter Drach.

⤚ 10 ⤙

Conrad von Megenberg's
Buch der Natur

ORTH of the Alps and the Pyrenees, science remained in the hands of the clergy much later than was the case in the south, as shown by the Arabic centers of learning in Moorish Spain and the lay school of medicine at Salerno. In England, such men as Roger Bacon, Grosseteste, Alexander Neckham, and Adelard of Bath were all clerics, and in France and Belgium, Vincent of Beauvais and Thomas de Cantimpré were members of monastic orders. In the Germanic areas the list was equally imposing: Hildegarde of Bingen was an Abbess, and Albertus Magnus and Conrad von Megenberg were Bishops.

Conrad was born in the small town of Megenberg near Schweinfurth around the year 1309. In his youth he studied the liberal arts at Erfurt and attended the University of Paris. There he became a Magister, afterwards teaching philosophy and theology from about 1329 to 1337. He then became director of the St. Stephen's School in Vienna, and in 1342, still a parish priest, he transferred to Ratisbon where he ad-

73

vanced to the position of Canon of the Cathedral. He died in
Ratisbon on April 14, 1374, and was buried in a Benedictine
nunnery there. During his lifetime he made one special
journey to the Papal Court at Avignon where, in 1357, he
defended the rights of a Benedictine abbey, that of St. Em-
meram, before the Roman Curia.

From the foregoing it is obvious that Conrad was both
well educated and competent, precisely the kind of man to
compose an encyclopedia for those who spoke only the common tongue. In this case it was a German dialect which was
then spoken in the Bavarian-Austrian borderland region.
His purpose was to advance the education of women and
the common people who were not learned in Latin. Though
some say it was written in Vienna, it must have been done
at Ratisbon, for he lived there at the reputed time of writing,
between 1349 and 1351.

Thanks to Conrad's efforts the *Natura rerum* of Thomas
de Cantimpré was given a new lease on life. Never printed
in its original form, Cantimpré's book nonetheless reached
the press in Conrad's altered version. This was an act of
preservation for which we can be grateful—there *are* occasions when plagiarism can be a virtuous deed.

Plagiarism, however, is too strong a word to use in this
case. Conrad merely reached for an authoritative work that
would be of use in bringing learning to his people, and he
added much of his own in the process. Cantimpré's book
had mentioned only 114 plants; Conrad added 59, making a
total of 173. The bulk of these, as extracted from Cantimpré,
had come from Platearius and the *Circa instans*. The rest
were gathered from a variety of authors, such as Avicenna,
Galen, Dioscorides, Isidore, and Conrad himself. Conrad's
own observations are generally prefaced with the phrase,
"Ich Megenberger waiz wol" (I, Megenberger, know well).
One of them relates to the dangers of eating mushrooms:
"Fungi are called Swammen," says Conrad. "There is also
one kind, which is called in Latin Boletos and in German

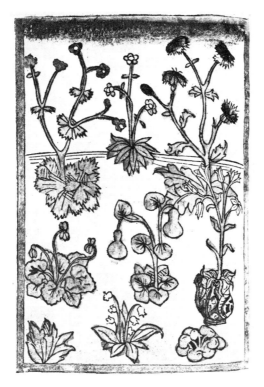

FIGURE 28. Plants. The first woodcut ever to present plants that were not mere ornaments nor parts of a landscape was this illustration for the 1475 edition of the *Buch der Natur*. It headed the fifth section (on plants) of Conrad von Megenberg's work. In all, 89 plants are discussed, and they form a most unsystematic arrangment that includes such diverse items as sage, sugar, mustard, lilies, violets, onions, crocus, and hops. (From Conrad von Megenberg's *Buch der Natur*. Augsburg, Hans Bämler, 1475. Original size 4 $^{15}/_{16}$" wide × 7 $^3/_{16}$" high.)

Pfifferling; they are poisonous and deadly, that I know well, for it happened at Wienn in Oesterreich, that one ate and drank of pfifferling and died." Someone had evidently mistaken a poisonous Boletus for the delectable *Boletus edulis*, an error that is still made today.

A few other glimpses of Conrad's times surface in his

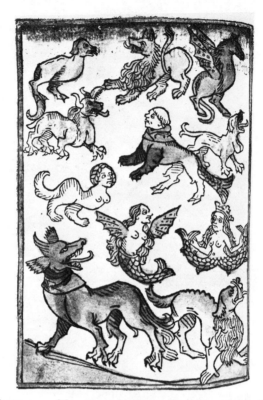

FIGURE 29. Monsters. No encyclopedia, since the days of Pliny, could dispense with its section on monsters. Here we find the treacherous monk-fish and the siren, both of whom lured victims into the sea, and an assorted lot of bipeds and quadrupeds. Many of these creatures seem to have been fathered in the minds of the Augsburg artists, who knew quite well that the odd and the exotic moved the curious into buying books that they would otherwise leave untouched. (From Conrad von Megenberg's *Buch der Natur.* Augsburg, Hans Bämler, 1475. Original size 5″ wide × 7 ³/₈″ high.)

writings. While discussing the plant Arum, he refers to its reputed power to drive away serpents and says that it was reported to grow in places where frogs and snakes dwell. But he goes on to say, "That know I, Megenberger, not, but I know this well, that the Master cultivated it in his Gärt-

leinn [little garden] before his sleep-chamber in Paris." Elsewhere he speaks of a comet, though it appears by his own
evidence tò have been a meteor, that crossed the sky in Paris
during 1337. It fell to the east in Germany, "and then shortly
after, I came here into German land, and there had been
many houses wrecked through Hungary, Austria, Bavaria,
and along the Main and Rhine." On another occasion he
saw a white rainbow, located at Riez near Nordlingen. He
also describes an earthquake at Villach in Carinthia, and the
ravages of the plague in Austria and Bavaria in 1349. Since
the earthquake had occurred a year earlier Conrad considered it to be the cause of the plague. He also informs us of
the appearance in Ratisbon, about 1350, of another plague to
mankind, the use of firearms.

The contents of the *Buch der Natur* are very similar to
those of Bartholomaeus Anglicus' *De proprietatibus rerum*
and, for that matter, to the even earlier *Physica* of Hildegarde of Bingen. Conrad's first section out of eight in the
Buch der Natur is on mankind, and includes 50 chapters on
anatomy, physiology, and the means of determining character through physical appearance and dreams. Book II concerns Heaven and the seven planets, astronomy, and meteorology, and has a total of 33 chapters. Book III is on zoology.
It lists 69 quadrupeds, 72 birds, 20 "sea-wonders" (including the crocodile, the sea-monk, and the mermaid), 29 fish
and the inevitable sea-serpent, 37 snakes, lizards, and reptiles, and 31 worms (under which heading he places bees,
obviously because of their larval stage). Book IV discusses
fruit, nut, and timber trees in 55 chapters, while devoting 29
more to aromatic trees. Book V describes some 89 herbs and
vegetables in as many chapters. Book VI discusses some 86
precious and semiprecious stones, while Book VII speaks of
10 kinds of metals. The eighth and final book is on the mar-
velous powers of streams and waters, with a section on
human monstrosities thrown in as a bonus. Of course in
Conrad's time such phenomena were regarded as signs from

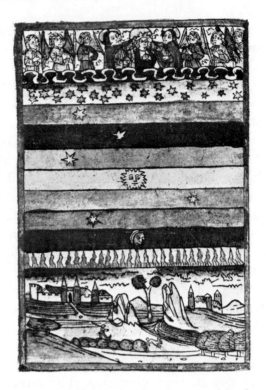

FIGURE 30. The Heavens. Conrad's second book, or
section, is on the heavenly bodies, the atmosphere,
weather, and such phenomena as the rainbow,
snow, and the causes of thunder and lightning. The
illustration shows the Macrocosm. At the top is the
Divine Sphere or Primum Mobile, then the fixed
stars and the paths of Saturn, Jupiter, Mars, the
Sun, Venus, Mercury, and the Moon. Below them is
the realm of the four elements, fire, air, water, and
earth, which surround and compose our world.
(From Conrad von Megenberg's *Buch der Natur.*
Augsburg, Hans Bämler, 1475. Original size 4 7/8"
wide × 7 1/4" high.)

the Deity, presaging changes in human affairs, and were
considered significant. In the medieval world everything
was a manifestation of God's will.

The *Buch der Natur* enjoyed great success in German-
speaking lands, and numerous manuscript copies were
made. Because of warfare and constantly shifting political

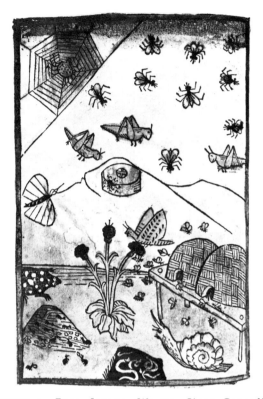

FIGURE 31. Bees, Insects, Worms. Since Conrad's book was largely derived from the work of Thomas Cantimpré it contained a lengthy passage on bees, Cantimpré having written a separate book on that subject. In the Middle Ages, insects, worms, snails, and other creatures that were not clearly birds, beasts, or fish presented some problems in classification. So did their products. Honey, for instance, comes under weather phenomena in Book II, right after the cause of mildew. (From Conrad von Megenberg's *Buch der Natur*. Augsburg, Hans Bämler, 1475. Original size 5" wide × 7 ⅛" high.)

boundaries, many of those manuscripts were either destroyed or had the details of their provenance thrown into confusion. Franz Pfeiffer, who edited a reprint of Conrad's work published in 1861, spoke of seventeen manuscripts in Munich, eight in Vienna, and three in Stuttgart, most of them from the 15th century. He mentions one manuscript

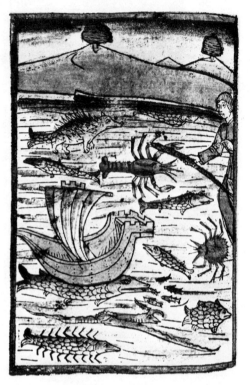

FIGURE 32. Sea Wonders. Since few landsmen had any idea of what creatures lived in the sea (nor did sailors and fishermen for that matter), there was ample scope for the imagination of story-tellers. A few of their inventions are seen here: the abydes, with its four feet, was born in the sea but later hunted on land; the serra carried a ship on its back until it sawed it through; the lobsterlike ceruleo, with claws sixty cubits in length, could pull elephants under water. (From Conrad von Megenberg's *Buch der Natur.* Augsburg, Hans Bämler, 1475. Original size 5" wide × 7 ³/₈" high.)

dated 1377, but no location is given. A great deal of water has gone under the bridge since then, and Conrad is not often discussed in print these days, so the present state of manuscript copies remains vague.

The printed editions of the *Buch der Natur* are a different matter, for they received expert treatment and loving attention from the printers of Augsburg. They issued six separate editions before 1500, and enlisted the talents of the famed woodblock cutters of Augsburg for their illustrations. Thanks to their imaginative and innovative designs, Conrad's *Buch der Natur* contains two firsts in the field of illustration. In the 1475 edition by Hans Bämler of Augsburg (who was himself a cutter of blocks), we find the first print of animals, and also the first printed representation of plants for a botanical or horticultural purpose, rather than an ornamental one. The plants in that cut antedate those of the *Herbarius latinus* by nine years, and the crude diagrammatic ones of Apuleius by six.

By reason of its present rarity and unavailability Conrad's book has fallen into obscurity. Even the industrious and generally accurate Pritzel, botany's bibliographer, listed Conrad's work as anonymous. But with improved bibliographies and modern methods of producing fine facsimiles, perhaps the same good fortune is in store for the *Buch der Natur* that once happened to Conrad himself. In 1358 he was stricken with a paralysis that fully possessed his feet and hands. Describing what happened, he says, "but I was made whole while prostrate before the altar of St. Echard in Ratisbon, while the alleluia 'O gemma pastoralis lucida' was sung, and as they followed with 'Salve splendor firmamenti.' " It is possible that Conrad's book, too, may once again "shine like a jewel."

BIBLIOGRAPHIC NOTES

Original manuscript not extant. Composed between 1349 and 1351, probably in Ratisbon.

Earliest manuscript: neither date nor location are known. A copy dated 1377 existed in 1861.

1st edition: 1475 at Augsburg by Hans Bämler. This was also the first illustrated edition.

Peter Schoeffer's *Herbarius Latinus*

OOK collectors have always cherished the *Herbarius latinus* for a number of reasons. For one thing, it contains 150 highly decorative woodcuts, which are now believed to have their models in the Salernitan series of illustrations. For another, it was printed by different printers at different places, and so exhibits some interesting variations. An enterprising bibliophile could make a career of tracking down every version, for there are known to be as many as eleven incunabula editions. Moreover, four variations occur in the first edition alone, but they are relatively minor and seem to be merely alterations made during the printing. The *Herbarius* also exists in Latin, Dutch, and Italian, with some editions carrying German, Dutch, or Flemish equivalents of the Latin plant names. In any case, there is ample variety for the book hunter, combined with the thrill of discovering very rare editions.

First printed at Mainz in 1484 by Peter Schoeffer, an associate of Gutenberg, the *Herbarius* was primarily intended

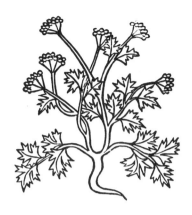

FIGURE 33. Coriander. Today coriander's principal use is as a spice and flavoring, but the *Herbarius Latinus* advised mixing it with warm vinegar and sempervivum to cure abscesses. It also shows a disagreement among the herbal authorities, for Galen and Serapion considered it warm in nature, while Dioscorides and Avicenna held it to be cold. The juice was used to stop nose-bleeds and, when mixed with violets, it was used to overcome drunkenness. (From the *Herbarius Latinus.* Vicenza, 1491. Original size 3 ⁷/₁₆" wide × 6 ¹/₁₆" high. Includes type *and* woodcut. Page size [margins included] 5 ¹/₄" wide × 7 ⁵/₈" high.)

for those who did not have access to physicians, or could not afford them. This is one of the reasons for the great number of illustrations, more than had accompanied any previous printed herbal. The illustrations have charm and attractiveness, but one would tend to doubt their usefulness for field identification, since they were rather schematic in style. In practice, however, most people were better acquainted with the appearance of their local flora than we are nowadays and needed only a sketchy indication, although an occasional mistake could prove fatal. Once they had the plant they sought in hand, the rest was a matter of following directions and hoping for the best.

The *Herbarius,* as it left Schoeffer's press, bore its name on the title page, the first time that such a thing had been done. Immediately following the name came the phrase *Moguntie impressus* (printed at Mainz), the date (1484), and the device of the printing firm of Fust and Schoeffer. A complication exists, however, for in the preface of the work its anonymous author specifically refers to the book as the "Aggregator practicus simplicibus." Later it picked up other aliases, such as "Tractatus virtutibus herbarum" (treatise on the virtues of herbs), "Herbolario volgare" (the common herbal), as well as "Herbarius Patavinus" (the Herbal of Pas-

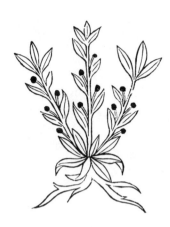

FIGURE 34. Madder. *Rubia tinctorum,* madder, forms the 121st chapter of the *Herbarius latinus.* It saw medicinal use as a
diuretic, for stomach ailments, hysteria,
and amenorrhea, and for complaints of the
liver and spleen. Its principal use, however, was as a dyestuff. From its roots,
rose, crimson, and other reddish colors
were derived, the different hues depending
on the means of extracting the dye and the
kind of mordant used to make it "set."
(From *Herbarius Latinus.* Vicenza, 1491.
Original size 3 ½" wide × 6 ¹/₁₆" high. Includes type *and* woodcut. Page size
[margins included] 5 ¼" wide × 7 ⁵/₈"
high.)

sau), and names of other towns it was printed in. Resolving
the confusion around the *Herbarius* has taken a century of
work, and has confounded many bibliographers who struggled to put the scanty data in order.

For a book that is straightforward and unpretentious in
its content, the *Herbarius* has managed to cause some sizable
bibliographic mistakes. One such error led to the persistent
belief that it was the work of Arnaldus de Villanova. His
only connection with the *Herbarius* was the use of his name
set below a woodcut that had been inserted as an illustration
just above the text of the preface. The cut was supposed to
show Arnaldus discussing plants with the Arabic physician,
Avicenna. The names of both men were set in type below
the cut, which was not misleading until the woodcut was
eliminated. Thereafter the names were allowed to stand as
the opening line of the book, thus seeming to indicate authorship. Not until bibliographers could set the 1491 edition
with the woodcut beside the later edition that had dropped
it, was the puzzle finally solved.

For a time the name *Herbarius* also led to confusion with
the *Herbarius zu Teutsch,* which was a name sometimes
given to another herbal masterpiece, *Der Gart.* What caused

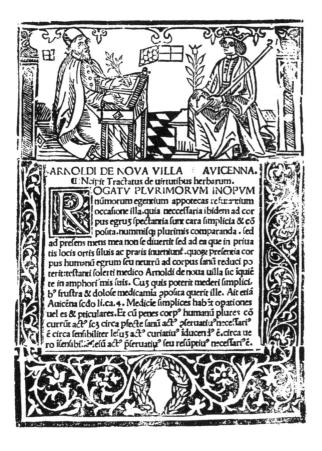

FIGURE 35. Arnaldus and Avicenna. The two gentlemen who grace the opening page of the 1491 edition of the *Herbarius Latinus* are not who they seem to be. Instead of being Arnaldus de Novavilla (Villanova) and Avicenna, as labelled here, they are Piero Crescentio and his patron Charles of Anjou in a woodcut for the *Opus ruralium commodorum* (issued in 1490 by the same printer and publisher). To compound the confusion, in subsequent editions of the *Herbarius* the woodcut was removed entirely, leaving the names to stand by themselves at the head of the text, and that gave birth to a persistent error about the authorship of the *Herbarius Latinus*. (From the *Herbarius Latinus*. Vicenza, 1491. Original size of page 5 ⁹/₁₆″ wide × 7 ¹/₂″ high.)

the confusion was the fact that the same printer, Peter Schoeffer, had produced both books. Today it is simple enough to tell those two herbals apart, for they have been carefully described, their pages have been counted and photographed, and they can easily be examined side by side in the larger collections. This of course was not the case in earlier times, when scholars frequently had access to no more than one or two editions and were often forced to rely on mere names and other insufficient data. The wonder is not that so many errors were made, but that so many were successfully corrected.

The *Herbarius* is divided into two major sections. The first contains descriptions and medicinal uses of 150 plants, all of which grew in Germany. Earlier works of the sort had never showed such specialization. This, in fact, is one of the reasons for believing the book was compiled on Schoeffer's order. There is further indication of a 15th-century origin in that it appears to have been meant for a German market only, for every one of the 150 plants of the main section bears the name in German as well as Latin. This practice, incidentally, carried over into some of the foreign editions, which used local Dutch, Flemish, and German dialects along with the Latin.

The *Herbarius* sold as well in Italy as it did in Germany, if not better. There its second section may have contributed to its success, for it was concerned with the materials of medicine that were commonly available in the shops of apothecaries and spice merchants. Through the use of the *Herbarius* the average man could easily find what drugs to use and purchase them in most towns. The second section has 96 chapters, though many of them are very brief. They deal with the following: laxatives; aromatics; fruits, seeds, and plants of garden and orchard; gums and resins; salts; minerals and stones; and a variety of animals and their products, such as goose-grease, cheese, honey, and ivory. Alphabetical order was adhered to in all parts of the *Her-*

barius, which made it simple to find each substance and the qualities ascribed to it.

Some notion of the information it gave is shown by the following quote taken from the chapter on coriander:

"Mark that the juice of this (coriander) mixed with juice of house-leek and warm vinegar is effective with abscesses. . . . In like manner coriander taken with vinegar soon after dining heavily prohibits vapors from rising to the head. . . . The juice of it with vinegar works against St. Anthony's fire (erysipelas). . . . Mark that the juice of coriander blown up the nostrils restrains nosebleed, and does the same when smelled or sniffed. . . . And coriander is effective in tremors of the heart when its powder is given with borage water."

The second section of the herbal is drawn from the *Pandects* of Matthaeus Sylvaticus, the *Circa instans,* Bartholomaeus Anglicus, Avicenna, and other writings. Among other things, we find that liquorice "and wine in a decoction is effective against coughing, and that liquorice chewed and retained on the tongue relieves thirst and rough dryness in the throat and stomach." Gum arabic was to be pounded, "and its powder mixed with the powder of dragon's blood [another resinous gum] and rose water is serviceable against fluxes of the blood or the menses." And in order "to rupture an abscess make a plaster of turpentine and wheat flour." For those who could afford it, since this item was *not* cheap, "Lapis lazuli . . . is effective against ailments of the heart if given with the juice of borage and the bone from the heart of a deer. And as it may be said briefly, it is effective against all the sufferings of melancholy." Melancholy in this case does not mean sadness, but a kind of madness thought to be caused by secretions from the spleen.

Within a few months of its release, the *Herbarius* was plagiarized in the German town of Speier, and in Louvain in Flanders. It was reproduced exactly, illustrations and all, but Schoeffer does not seem to have made any objection. After

all, most of the text of the *Herbarius* had been taken from
Vincent of Beauvais (without acknowledgment), along with
condensed extracts from other authors. The *Herbarius*, for all
its success, may have been only a trial run for a more ambitious publishing project, perhaps thus accounting for
Schoeffer's indifference regarding it. Schoeffer's more ambitious project was one of the most famous herbals ever
printed, *Der Gart der Gesundheit* (*The Garden of Good Health*),
and is the subject of the next chapter.

BIBLIOGRAPHIC NOTES

No manuscript or prototype known to exist. The work may very
well have been an original compilation constructed in
Schoeffer's printing establishment.

1st edition: 1484 at Mainz by Peter Schoeffer. Four variants are
known to exist, but are not regarded as separate editions,
merely as alterations during the printing run.
2nd edition: 1484 at Speier by J. and C. Hist.
3rd edition: 1484 at Kuilenburg by Jan Veldener.
4th edition: 1484 at Louvain by Jan Veldener.
5th edition: 1485–86 at Louvain by Jan Veldener.
6th edition: 1485 at Passau by Johann Petri.
7th and 8th editions: 1486 at Passau by Johann Petri.
9th edition: 1486 at Paris by Jean Bonhomme.
10th edition: 1491 at Vicenza by Leonardus Achates of Basle and
Gulielmus of Pavia.
11th edition: 1499 at Venice by Simon Bevilacqua.
Last edition: 1565 at Venice by Francesco de Leno.

Since the Herbarius has had a tangled bibliographic history the
above list of the incunabula editions may help to keep the
present record straight.

⊷ 12 ⊶

Peter Schoeffer's *Der Gart*

NE year after the resounding success of his *Herbarius,* Schoeffer set ajar the gates of modern scientific publishing with the printing of *Der Gart der Gesundheit.* While it retained much that was as medieval as anything in the *Herbarius,* or in Bartholomaeus Anglicus, it also made some significant advances. For instance, for the first time Latin and Greek were abandoned and the book spoke to its readers in their own vernacular German. This does not mean, however, that the language is easy for readers of modern German to comprehend. The text is in a Bavarian dialect, as shown by the following sample about an unexpected property of bituminous coal: "Eyn meister Enax genant spricht in synem lapidario das diss sy cyn edel gestein syner dogent halben went er benympt alle dufels melancoly" ("A master named Enax says in his Book of Stones that this is a gemstone that has power to turn away all demons and melancholy from virgins [who carry it]"). The content in this case may not seem progressive, but at least the restrictions caused by the classical languages had disappeared once and for all.

Another innovation was the obvious return to nature as

89

a source for the botanical illustrations of *Der Gart*. No work
on plants, since the days of Crateuas in the 1st century B.C.,
had seen fit to seek out truth of form by observing and
drawing nature's own productions. Out of the 379 woodcuts
designed for *Der Gart*, some 65 are faithful renditions clearly
based on the plants themselves, a very high proportion for
the time. A great deal of their verity, in the opinion of Dr.
Arnold Klebs, is the result of using larger woodcuts; in this
instance they averaged about five by seven inches. The
larger dimensions permitted inclusion of more identifying
detail than was possible with the usual blocks, which were
about half that size. In subsequent editions of *Der Gart*
printed by other publishers, that advantage was sacrificed to
greater economy and higher profit through the use of
smaller cuts.

The remaining 314 illustrations for *Der Gart* carried on
the traditions established by the Salernitan series of depictions. Schoeffer's exact source for these has not been found
as yet, but it is known that he had a sizable collection of
manuscripts at his printing establishment in Mainz. That, as
a matter of fact, was a common practice among early
printers. After all, if you were going to print a copy of Pliny
or the *Proprietatibus rerum* you had to have an accurate
model.

The early printer's task of reproducing the great works
of all ages had once been the province of the scriptoria of
abbeys and monasteries. As interest arose in secular learning, and universities were established to provide it, the sta-

FIGURE 36. Frontispiece of *Der Gart*. This frontispiece presents a gathering
of the most notable herbalists of all ages. Only the central three in the
foreground can be identified with any degree of certainty. They are probably the Roman, Pliny (at the left), the Greek, Dioscorides (in the center),
and either Mesue or Serapion, both Arabic (on the right). The blank
shield hanging over them was often used for adding the book owner's
initials or coat of arms in ink or color. (From *Der Gart*. Mainz, Peter
Schöffer, 1485. Reduced from original size of frontispiece, 7 9/16" wide ×
11" high.)

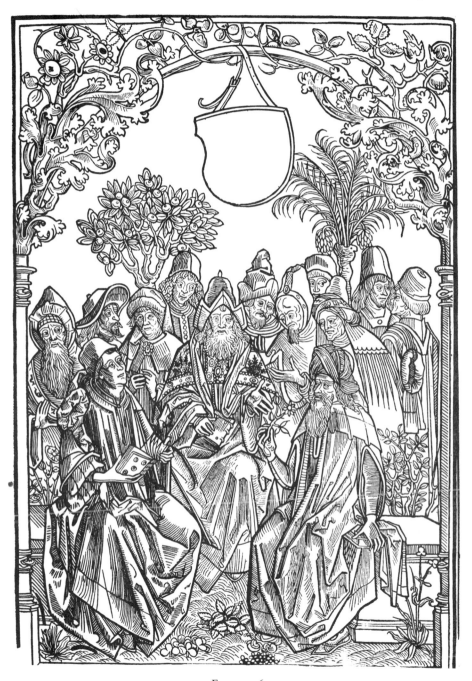

FIGURE 36.

tionarii and librarii came into being. They produced, sold, or rented manuscripts for the use of students and magisters in the great schools of Paris, Bologna, and other centers. The entire book trade was closely regulated and the privileges of each group were carefully legislated. Parchment dealers could sell their wares in certain places at certain times and were bound to give preference to special sections of the community, such as the magisters or the stationarii (stationers) of the universities.

What profits there were from the book trade went to the parchment suppliers and the booksellers, and they were often considerable. A Bible could cost as much as 10,000 francs in an ordinary, undecorated, unilluminated state. The scribes who did such work were not highly paid, however; one 15th-century record mentions a sum of £200 as payment for five years' work by two scribes who transcribed *Parsival*. Authors, of course, fared even worse. Once their manuscript began to circulate there was no means of retaining control of it, nor of profiting from its popularity. They were, accordingly, either of independent means or able to attract patronage. Some were engaged or ordered to compose a work that the Church or State deemed needful for its own purposes. Printing altered all of that, reducing the price of books by as much as four-fifths, and made knowledge more readily available.

Schoeffer was among the first to realize the changed order of things. Not only did he decide to publish in vernacular German to reach a wider audience, he also moved his publishing headquarters to Frankfurt while retaining his printing press in Mainz. Moreover, he set up branches in Paris and Angers to distribute his publications, thus operating internationally, as his heirs would still be doing in the mid-15th century when they commissioned Venetian presses to print books for them. Another step in the direction of modern publishing was his realization that the usefulness of a work could be improved by providing adequate

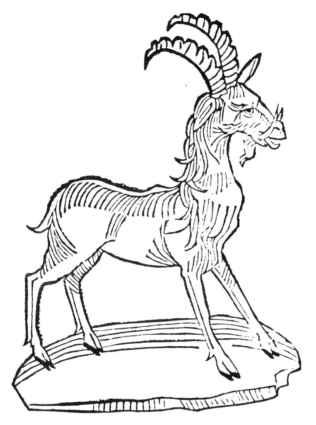

FIGURE 37. Musk Deer. This Asiatic animal's scent-glands were highly valued by the ancients and the people of the Middle Ages. The scent was synthesized in modern times, but only after the creature became almost extinct. The real animal does not look nearly as belligerent as shown here, but if it did it might have intimidated a few hunters at least. (From *Der Gart*. Mainz, P. Schöffer, 1485. Original size 4 $^1/_8$" wide × 5 $^9/_{16}$" high.)

indices. *Der Gart* offered its readers an alphabetical listing of every disease or ailment then known, and under each such heading made reference to chapters that discussed remedies, pointing out particular paragraphs that had special pertinence. The medicinal simples themselves were listed alphabetically as well as by their chapter numbers. Unlike other incunabula, *Der Gart* did not frustrate its users in their search for particulars.

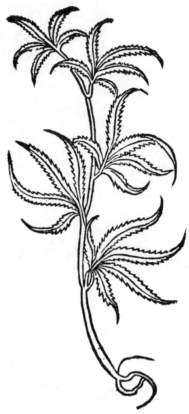

FIGURE 38. Cannabis. Canapus or Hanff, as *Der Gart* called it, was considered hot and dry in the second degree. It was prescribed for distended
stomachs, dropsy, pains in the anal region, and as a plaster for boils and
carbuncles. Applied to wounds it relieved pain, and a decoction of its
roots and seeds mixed with white lead and oil of roses was used to treat
erysipelas. Only when its vapors were employed to ease headache did it
come close to its modern use as a hallucinogen, for Canapus is medieval
Latin for *Cannabis sativa,* our "pot," "marijuana," or "grass." (From *Der
Gart.* Mainz, P. Schöffer, 1485. Original size 4 ³/₄" wide × 6 ¹¹/₁₆" high.)

There are 435 chapters in *Der Gart,* the bulk of them
concerned with plants, but a few minerals and some animal
products are also included, and there is an additional section on uroscopy. Uroscopy was a means of diagnosis used
throughout the Middle Ages in which the physician exam-

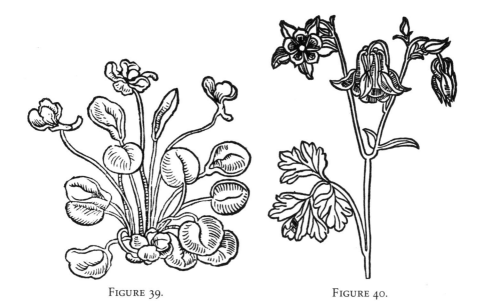

FIGURE 39.   FIGURE 40.

FIGURE 39. Viola. The name of the artist who did the better drawings in *Der Gart* is not known with certainty, but Erhard Reuwich has been suggested as a strong possibility. He was active in Mainz about 1485 and had a similar style. Unlike many other woodcuts of the era, those in *Der Gart* were often based on nature (as was this picture of violets) rather than on patterns created earlier to serve as artist's aids. Violets, mixed with flour paste, were used to treat inflamed eyes, mouths, or stomachs, and to relieve intestinal pains, among other things. (From *Der Gart*. Mainz, P. Schöffer, 1485. Original size 4 ³/₄" wide × 4 ³/₈" high.)

FIGURE 40. Columbine. Although listed in the herbals, columbine had relatively little use medicinally. The leaves were sometimes used in a lotion for sore throat, or the seeds were mixed with wine and saffron to relieve the liver. But it was generally regarded as a garden plant. Its pendant flowers, which were thought to resemble doves, caused it to become a symbol of the Holy Ghost. (From *Der Gart*. Mainz, Peter Schöffer, 1485. Original size 4 ³/₄" wide × 5 ¹/₄" high.)

ined his patient's urine by holding a flask of it to the light. He searched for color, particles, suspended cloudiness at various levels, and sediment. The flask, called a matula, was marked off to aid the process. Some physicians claimed to be able to tell the age, sex, and general condition of a person without recourse to any other data. The system remained in use through the 17th century, and is pictured in some of the genre paintings of Gerard Dou and Adrian van Ostade.

Der Gart was, in every respect, a noble work that included all the medical knowledge of its time. It has no known author and, like its predecessor the *Herbarius*, is thought to be a compilation made to Schoeffer's specifications. A physician of the day, Johan von Cube, is quoted in Chapter 76. Discussing the styptic properties of Armenian bole, an astringent earth, he says "eyn gewisse artzney dicke mail versuecht an vil enden von mir Meister Johann von Cube" ("A true doctor coated muslin with it and tried it to end [bleeding] by me Master Johann von Cube"). On the basis of this passage he is sometimes credited with authorship of the work. It is much more likely that, as Town Physician of Frankfurt (where Schoeffer had kept his publishing headquarters since 1479, the press itself being at Mainz), von Cube was called upon to edit or verify the text of *Der Gart*.

Its tone and intent were lofty, as can be seen in these words from the prologue: "Many a time and oft have I bethought within myself of the wondrous works of the Shaper of the Universe. . . . While considering these matters I likewise recalled that the Shaper of Nature, Who has set us amidst such perils, has granted us a remedy with all manner of herbs, animals, and sundry other created things. . . . I thank Thee, O Shaper of heaven and earth . . . that Thou hast granted to me grace of revealing this treasure, which has until now lain hidden and buried from the sight of common men."

Some of the "common men" were quick to take advantage of a good thing. Within five months of *Der Gart*'s publication Johann Schoensperger of Augsburg had plagiarized it exactly, merely reversing the illustrations. From then until 1502 he repeated the outrage eight more times, but used cuts of a smaller size. Nor was he alone, for there were four others who profited illicitly from Schoeffer's labors. All that can be said to mitigate their offense is that they increased the incunabula editions of *Der Gart* prodigiously, and hastened its distribution throughout Germany, Switzerland, and the Netherlands. As a result, *Der Gart*'s chances for survival were greatly enhanced.

BIBLIOGRAPHIC NOTES

No manuscript known to exist.

1st edition: March 28, 1485, at Mainz by Peter Schoeffer.
2nd edition: August 22, 1485, at Augsburg by Johann Schoensperger.
3rd edition: June 5, 1486, at Augsburg by Hanns (Johann) Schoensperger.
4th edition: 1486 at Strassburg by Johann Grüninger.
5th edition: 1486/87 at Basel by Michael Furter.
6th edition: March 7, 1487, at Augsburg by Hanns Schoensperger.
7th edition: March 31, 1487, at Ulm by Conrad Dinckmut.
8th edition: 1488 at Augsburg by [Johann] Schoensperger.
9th edition: December 15, 1488, at Augsburg by Hanns Schoensperger.
10th edition: 1489 at Strassburg by Johann Grüninger.
11th edition: 1492 at Lübeck by Steffan Arndes (a translation into Low German).
12th edition: August 13, 1493, at Augsburg by Hanns Schoensperger. There is a variant of this, same date and place, but with "alterhandt" instead of "allerhandt" in the title.
13th edition: May 10, 1496, at Augsburg by Hanns Schoensperger.
14th edition: May 13, 1499, at Augsburg by Hanns Schoensperger.

This is the complete list of incunabula editions known to Klebs's *Incunabula Scientifica et Medica,* and to Nissen's *Botanische Buchillustration.*
All editions are illustrated.

Arbolayre, or *Le Grant Herbier*

HERE is probably no book in all of herbal literature which has caused greater bibliographic confusion than *Le Grant Herbier.* In regard to problems of anonymity, uncertain dates, fictitious personalities, and dubious editions, *Le Grant Herbier* leads all contenders for the championship of chaos. Like many other medieval herbals its author is anonymous and, like the *Herbarius* and *Der Gart,* it had more than one name. In its first edition it was known as *Arbolayre*—a pleasant, brief, and lyrical title. But it was promptly dropped in favor of *Le Grant Herbier,* the name it bore from the second through all succeeding editions. It also had a plentiful supply of printers—at least six of them—and was printed in Besançon, Paris, and Lyons. Another difficulty was that the date of issue was seldom included, so the history of the book could not be reconstructed without reconstructing the careers of its printers.

Moreover, its illustrations are based on a series of smaller woodcuts created for *Der Gart.* The book also borrowed from the *Circa instans,* for 264 of the 474 chapters in *Le Grant Herbier* are taken from the famed Salernitan work. This, of course, led to the statement by some scholars that the *Circa instans* exists in its fullest state only as *Le Grant Herbier,* and that the two are merely long and short versions of the same work. What, precisely, was the rationale behind two states of one book is a question that has never been satisfactorily answered. If it meant reducing a large compendium to digest form there would be an obvious advantage, but in this instance some 201 chapters are dropped in their entirety. Such a truncation might be conceivable in a literary work, but the *Circa* was concerned with pharmacy and medicinal plants. It is difficult to see what standard was applied in the exclusion of some chapters and the retention of others, since all were pertinent.

Before entering on the complexities that have grown out of the *Circa* and *Grant Herbier* relationship, it may be best to give a brief summation of the French herbal itself. Its purpose was to inform both laymen and physicians about medicinal preparations and how to administer them. In this it resembled the *Circa,* the *Herbarius,* and *Der Gart.* Most versions of *Le Grant Herbier* are about 474 chapters in length, but some 16th-century printings have 500 or more. Its only translation was into English as the *Grete Herball,* which differs frequently from its model. For example, the prologue of the *Grete Herball* resembles that of *Der Gart,* whereas the prologue of *Le Grant Herbier* resembles that of the *Circa instans.*

Le Grant Herbier was repeatedly printed in France, where it received heavy use by owners who seem to have subjected it to more than average wear. Pages are frequently missing, while others have been chewed by rodents or drilled through by bookworms. Complete and undamaged copies are almost unheard of. The work is also excessively rare in either 15th- or 16th-century editions. No more than five copies of its first edition, c. 1486–88 (when it was called *Arbolayre*), are known to exist. Quite naturally the foregoing factors of rarity and incompleteness have greatly impeded proper study of the work.

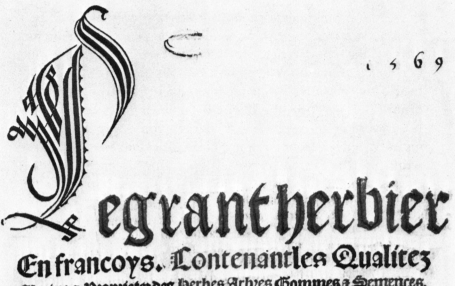

1 5 6 9

Le grant herbier

En francoys. Contenant les Qualitez

Uertus & Proprietez des Herbes Arbres Gommes & Semences.
Extraict de plusieurs traictez De medecine Comme de Aui-
cenne de Ralis de Constantin de Isaac de Plataire Se-
lon le commum vsaige. Et a este nouuellement
Imprime a Paris par Iaques Nyuerd.

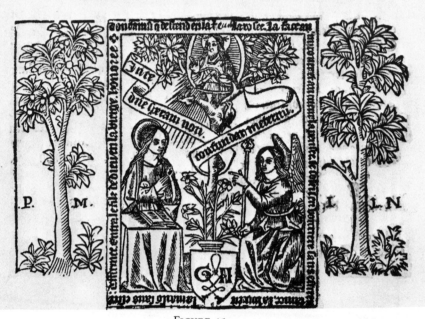

FIGURE 41.

Unresolved questions still surround *Le Grant Herbier*. We do not know who its compiler was (it consists of extracts from a number of works), nor when and why it was first put together. Clearing away those mysteries is a matter for continued research into the origins of *Le Grant Herbier*, and its problems need not have concerned us here except for the fact that its history became linked with that of the *Circa instans*. That unlucky circumstance came about in 1886 when Giulio Camus published a bibliographic discovery he had made in the Regia Biblioteca Estense, Modena, Italy.

Camus, in the course of comparing a 15th-century manuscript in Latin called *Tractatus Herbarum* (Codex 993) with a 15th-century manuscript in French titled *Secres de Salerne* (Codex 28), came to the correct conclusion that *both* texts contained the same material found in the printed *Le Grant Herbier*. He promptly claimed that they represented the original text of that work. Whether or not that is the case is outside our purpose here, and all would have been well if he had confined himself to that statement. But Camus went on to add that those texts also represented a larger version of the *Circa instans*, which he termed the complete state of that work. Confusion has existed ever since, and even trapped the ever careful historian of science, George Sarton.

Possibly what led Camus astray was the fact that almost all of the text found in printed copies of the *Circa* is translated word for word and incorporated into *Le Grant Herbier*. The printed *Circa* has 273 chapters, 264 of which appear in

FIGURE 41. Title page of *Le Grant Herbier*. The scene of the Annunciation appears on this title page because the printer had it on hand and thought it would make a decorative addition. In a sense it also suggests that medicinal treatment of disease is akin to mankind's redemption. Despite the presence of the number 1569 (added in ink by a former owner) the edition is undated, having been printed anytime between 1521 and 1544. *Le Grant Herbier* is the ancestor of the English *Grete Herball*, and is an expanded version of the 12th-century manuscript *Circa instans*. (From *Le Grant Herbier*. Paris, Jacques Nyverd, after 1520. Original size 7 $^{11}/_{16}$" wide × 11" high.)

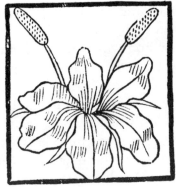

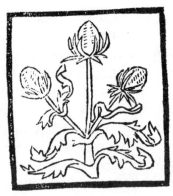

FIGURE 42.   FIGURE 43.

FIGURE 42. Plantain. A weed found by every wayside, Plantain was used from ancient times for any number of ills, sores, and wounds. It was also known as Arnoglosson (i.e., lamb's tongue), Waybread (a corruption of Waybrod, so named from its habit of growing by roadsides), and White Man's Foot (since it sprang up wherever white settlers in America walked). It cleared the chest and cured wounds, gout, intermittent fevers, and the bites of scorpions and spiders. (From *Le Grant Herbier*. Paris, J. Nyverd, after 1520. Original size 2 $^{7}/_{16}$" wide × 2 $^{9}/_{16}$" high.)

FIGURE 43. Fuller's teasle. The illustrations in *Le Grant Herbier* were debased adaptations of those from the *Herbarius latinus* and *Der Gart*, and the typography left much to be desired, since it often closed up spaces between words or carried them on to the next line without any indication. Fuller's teasle, seen here, was principally used to raise the nap on wool, but had some slight medicinal value, and was used in clysters, in suppositories, and to stop fluxes of blood. (From *Le Grant Herbier*. Paris, J. Nyverd, after 1520. Original size 2 $^{5}/_{16}$" wide × 2 $^{5}/_{8}$" high.)

Le Grant Herbier, but the French work has over 200 additional ones and generally averages 480 chapters in its various editions. Camus assumed that the extra chapters, not found in the printed *Circa instans*, must have belonged to it at an earlier time.

Against the notion put forward by Camus are these facts:

1. Both manuscripts upon which he based his idea of a longer version of the *Circa instans* are from the 15th

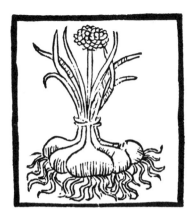

FIGURE 44. Cepe (Onion). Onions once served many other purposes than merely topping hamburger patties. *Le Grant Herbier* prescribed them for the bites of mad dogs, maladies that came of cold causes, and even for hemorrhoids, among many other things. Red onions were considered to be more styptic or drying in their action than the white ones. (From *Le Grant Herbier*. Paris, J. Nyverd, after 1520. Original size 2 $^{5}/_{16}$" wide × 2 $^{5}/_{8}$" high.)

century, 300 years later than the composition of the *Circa,* c. 1140.

2. No manuscript entitled *Circa instans* of more than 273 chapters (the amount found in its 1st edition) has ever been discovered.

3. The two earliest manuscripts now known of the *Circa* (c. 1190 and c. 1200–25) contain 258 and 260 chapters respectively. Those numbers are closer to the 273 of the printed *Circa* than the nearly 500 of *Le Grant Herbier.*

4. *Secres de Salerne,* which Camus rightly regarded as being synonymous with *Le Grant Herbier,* was popular in France and circulated widely there in manuscript. Other countries do not seem to know it or remark about it. It seems to be of French, *not* Salernitan, origin.

5. The reference to Salerno in *Secres de Salerne* indicates the source of the contents. The title, however, makes no mention of *Circa instans*. Avoidance of the name *Circa instans*, which was internationally recognized, would seem to indicate that its compiler considered it a different book.

6. The inclusion of chapters from *Circa instans* is not, in itself, proof that other chapters also came from that work.

7. The title page of *Le Grant Herbier* (Camus's *Secres de Salerne* and his candidate for the larger, complete state of *Circa instans*) says that it is composed of many extracts from Avicenna, Rhazes, Isaac, Platearius, and Constantine. But Avicenna, remained untranslated and unknown to Europeans, including Platearius (author of the *Circa*), until c. 1180, about 40 years after the *Circa* was written. Obviously Avicenna could not have furnished any of the material for the extra chapters of the supposed larger, "complete" *Circa*.

8. Nowhere does the surviving Salernitan literature support the contention that a longer version of *Circa instans* ever existed.

The foregoing leads us to these conclusions:

1. The only valid connection between *Circa instans* and *Le Grant Herbier* is that the latter availed itself of the text of the former.

2. There is no foundation for the theory that the *Circa instans* ever existed in a longer version, and no documentary proof of such a work has ever been brought forward.

3. *Le Grant Herbier*, contrary to Camus's statement that it is the *complete* text of *Circa instans*, says that it contains extracts from Arabic authors who had no part in the composition of the *Circa*. Extra material (beyond

that extracted from the *Circa*) should be considered as coming from the Arabic sources mentioned.

The theory of Camus that a longer *Circa instans* was reduced from about 480 chapters to 273 or less goes against the normal pattern of herbal evolution, which is that of gradual growth. It is unfortunate that he ever linked *Le Grant Herbier* and the *Circa,* clouding their true relationship and creating a bibliographic confusion that has persisted ever since 1886. The contention that *Le Grant Herbier* represents a complete text of the *Circa instans* must be viewed with the greatest suspicion and regarded as an unproven hypothesis.

BIBLIOGRAPHIC NOTES

Manuscript copies: Codex 993, Biblioteca Estense, Modena, Italy (a 15th-century Latin manuscript entitled *Tractatus Herbarum*). Codex 28, Biblioteca Estense (a French manuscript called *Secres de Salerne;* Camus calls this a 15th-century manuscript, but the c. 1790 catalogue of the Library says 14th century).

Codex 993 (above) contains the text of *Circa instans* plus an additional 200 or more extracts from the writings of Avicenna, Rhazes, Isaac, and others. Codex 28 (above) contains the same material plus 8 extra chapters. Both codices are almost identical with the text of the printed *Le Grant Herbier,* and both are illustrated. For further details see *L'Opera Salernitana "Circa instans" ed il testo primitivo del "Grant Herbier en Francoys."* Modena, 1886.

1st edition: c. 1486–88 by Pierre Metlinger at Besançon. The illustrations come from Johann Grüninger's edition of *Der Gart.*
2nd edition: c. 1498 by Pierre Le Caron at Paris. Illustrations same as in first edition.
3rd edition: c. 1498–1500 by Pierre Le Caron at Paris. The last of the incunabula editions. Illustrated as editions above. Over 20 16th-century editions are recorded. All have smaller, cruder versions of the same illustrations set in black-line frames. All are quite rare.

Jacob Meydenbach's *Hortus Sanitatis*

LTHOUGH it was published in 1491, just one year before Columbus discovered America, the *Hortus* still retains the flavor of the Middle Ages. Its appearance marked the end of an era in medicine and botany, for it was the last work to be derived in its entirety from earlier herbal authorities and to deal with Old World medicaments only. As is the case with *Der Gart*, the *Herbarius*, and *Le Grant Herbier*, it has no known author, but from internal evidence it seems to be a compilation made for (or by) Jacob Meydenbach of Mainz, its printer-publisher. In the epilogue he claims credit for its production, and may well have been responsible for more than the mere printing of it.

As a kind of valedictory to the medieval era the *Hortus* provides a truly grand finale. More copious than any of the earlier herbals, it has 1,066 chapters plus a treatise on uroscopy. Each chapter has an illustration at its head, and there are seven full-page woodcuts as well, making a total of 1,073 pictures. It is doubtful that any present-day work, other than a multi-volumed one, offers such a great number of illustrations.

Prior to the publication of the *Hortus* there had been a steady increase in the number of pictures used to illustrate books. Meydenbach's decision to incorporate so many woodcuts in his first major publication was, therefore, part of an established trend and affirmation of it. Afterwards only one herbal, that of Bock, dared to dispense with illustrations, but corrected the omission in its second edition.

The illustrations were a considerable expense for Meydenbach, despite the fact that those of plants were largely based on the small designs done for *Der Gart* in Schönsperger's and Grüninger's editions. He had to commission about 100 more plant cuts because the *Hortus* had 530 plant chapters while Der Gart had only 409. Meydenbach also had to provide original designs for 536 other chapters on animals, birds, fish, and minerals, plus seven full-page woodcuts. The format of his book was ample, and the type was spaced to allow for highly attractive and well-balanced pages. This required more paper, and it is doubtful that Meydenbach made much of a profit on his endeavor.

The *Hortus* was the first printed book to discuss so extensively the other kingdoms of nature. Since it had no rivals in those areas it was reprinted again and again by a variety of printers in different locations. There were three incunabula editions by Johann Prüss, one by Antoine Vérard, and some 16th-century printings in Venice, Strassburg, Frankfurt, and Paris. The complete work is generally in Latin, but French, English, German, and Dutch translations do exist. Many of the translations, however, include the tracts on zoology and minerals only, since those sections were far and away the most popular with the nonmedical public. One of these abbreviated versions, *The Noble Lyfe and Natures of Man,* has the distinction of being one of the world's rarest books. There are only two extant copies, both of which are in England. For centuries it was unrecognized

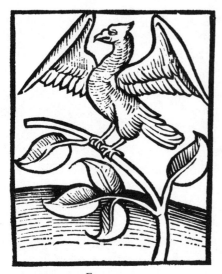 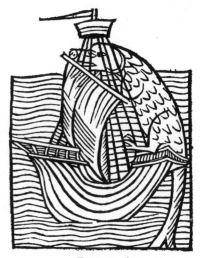

FIGURE 45.   FIGURE 46.

FIGURE 45. Caladrius. The Caladrius was a most unusual bird of purest white. If it gazed at a sick man from the foot of his bed he would recover, but if it averted its eyes the case was hopeless. In the former case it supposedly inhaled the illness and then rose to the sun where the sickness was burnt out, and the patient made whole again. Its history goes back to the legends first given currency in the *Physiologus,* a Greek work compiled at Alexandria about A.D. 200. (From the *Hortus Sanitatis.* Strassburg, J. Prüss, c. 1497. Original size 2 ¹/₂″ wide × 3 ¹/₈″ high.)

FIGURE 46. Pistris. The huge marine animal shown weighing down a vessel was generated out of a series of scribal errors. Here it is labelled Pistris and was said to interfere with ships in the Bay of Biscay, with Pliny cited as the authority. But according to Pliny, Pistris was really Pristis, a shark of the Indian Ocean, while the sperm-whale (Physeter) was the danger lurking off the French coast. (From the *Hortus Sanitatis.* Strassburg, J. Prüss, c. 1497. Original size 2 ¹/₂″ wide × 3 ¹/₈″ high.)

due to its altered title, but thanks to a clue discovered by Mr. Noel Hudson in the description of a woodcut, it was properly identified in 1954.

In addition to providing an innovative guide to zoological and minerological subjects, the index to the *Hortus* exceeded even that of *Der Gart* in the detail of its listings. The user had only to determine what ailment he wished to heal—for instance, Alopiciam (falling hair), or Yliaca passio (twisting pains in the small intestines)—and the index listed the location of the cure by chapter and line. This was accomplished by a matching set of letters, those in the index being paired with others in the margins of the text.

Since 1491 the *Hortus*, despite its numerous printings, has grown steadily rarer. A prime copy of Meydenbach's first edition cost about $200 at the beginning of this century. By the 1960s it had soared to $10,000, and current prices exceed that figure by a healthy margin. Back in 1501 Henry VII of England purchased a copy in French translation for six pounds, but that sum is a bit deceptive since the pound had at that time a purchasing power of about 130 of our 1976 dollars.

In addition to its comprehensiveness and rarity the *Hortus* had another notable feature, it was fashion-conscious. While depictions of plants, beasts, and minerals remained much the same over the centuries, costumes and styles underwent constant change. The Mainz 1491 edition showed clothing typical of 15th-century Germany, but the edition that came from a Strassburg printshop showed all persons in the genre scenes wearing proper Alsatian dress. In the Venetian edition, Italian garments are worn in woodcuts that are otherwise alike.

Throughout the *Hortus* every quote is identified as to source or author. The authorities cited form a most imposing list: Dioscorides, Albertus Magnus, Rhazes, Galen, Pliny, Mesue, and many others such as Palladius, Haly Abbas, Cassius Felix, Almansor, Isidore of Seville, and Virgil. The book makes a great show of being a medical work (such books sold very well in the 15th century), but actually its element of the fabulous and its delightful pictorial content were the real attractions. One cannot deny the charm of its content: "Anise has an odor that is goodly and strong. And that which comes out of the Island of Crete is the best. And after that the sort that is from Babylon. . . . It may be employed in a fumigation of the nostrils and so will ease an

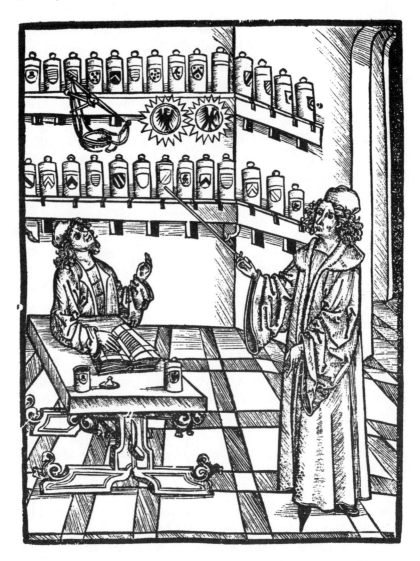

FIGURE 47. Physician in apothecary shop. Here is shown a 15th-century apothecary's shop with its jars of medicinal simples ranged upon the shelves. The physician is indicating which herbal substances he wants, and he probably will not be disappointed if the seals displayed have any official meaning. Standards for pharmacies and pharmacists were already being established. (From the *Hortus Sanitatis*. Strassburg, J. Prüss, c. 1497. Original size 5 $^5/_{16}$" wide × 7 $^1/_4$" high.)

aching head. For an aching of the ears it may be used with oil of roses to lessen the pains, and yet again to take away the griefs of a belly stuffed with wind" (my translation). Or when speaking of the remarkable virtues of the lodestone, a magnetic rock referred to as Lapis magnetis, the *Hortus* observes that it may be used as a marital compass as well as a navigational one. "And when this stone is placed beneath the head of a faithful woman she is, on the instant, moved to open her arms to her husband as she is overcome with the weight of sleep. Yet if she be an adultress then through evil dreams she will suffer such fear and trembling, beyond all measure, that it is said she will fall out of the marriage bed." If he had a copy of the *Hortus* and a handy magnet, the average 15th-century man, it seems, had no need for a marriage counselor.

BIBLIOGRAPHIC NOTES

No manuscript is known to exist.

1st edition: 1491 by Jacob Meydenbach at Mainz. 1,066 illustrations in text plus 7 full-page woodcuts, with a total of 1,073. Full-page cuts are (1) 3 doctors seated, 6 standing; (2) 3 men at right and animals in foreground; (3) 2 men seated amidst variety of birds; (4) 2 men standing at a harbor's edge, fish, mermaid and merman in water; (5) jeweller's shop with 12 people; (6) apothecary's shop with 9 figures, including 2 quarreling boys; (7) a patient in bed, one on crutches, another seated, 2 other figures in center, plus a man, woman, child, and infant in foreground, totaling 9 figures. Text: Prohemium; Herbs, 530 chapters; Animals, 164 chapters; Birds, 122 chapters; Fish, 106 chapters; Stones, 144 chapters; Treatise on Urines; Index of diseases and remedies; Alphabetical indices to Herbs, Animals, Birds, Fish, and Stones.

2nd edition: c. 1497 by Johann Prüss at Strassburg. The edition bears no printed date. One copy has a written date of purchase: November 12, 1497. 1,066 text cuts copied from Meydenbach, but details and costumes are changed. There are 3 full-page cuts: (1) teacher and students; (2) apothecary and physician; (3) skeleton. This edition formed the model for the succeeding Latin editions. Cut of skeleton borrowed from Johann Grüninger *after* July 1497, Prüss's edition on sale by November 12, 1497; therefore printed between beginning of August and end of October, 1497.

3rd edition: c. 1497 by Johann Prüss at Strassburg. Difficult to distinguish from 2nd edition. Slight rearrangement of text, and woodcuts not as fresh as the first printing. No date.

4th edition: c. 1499 by Johann Prüss at Strassburg. Block of apothecary and physician reduced in height. A page made up of four small cuts from the text precedes the Tract on Animals. Treatise on Urines has illustration of patient in bed attended by 3 doctors; borrowed from H. Brunschwig's *Cirurgia*. No date.

5th edition: c. 1500 by Antoine Vérard at Paris. 2-volume edition in French. Very rare. Last incunabula edition.

Two important 16th-century editions:

1511 edition by Bernardinus Benalius and Joannes Tacuinus de Cereto de Tridino at Venice. Latin text, but first edition of Hortus to be printed in Italy. Contains Galen's "De facile acquisibilibus."

1517 edition by Renatus Beck at Strassburg. This reproduces the Prüss editions because Beck was the successor at the Prüss establishment. It also has a title page attributed to Urs Graf.

Subsequent 16th-century editions printed the full text on only two occasions:

c. 1529 edition by Philippe le Noir at Paris. French translation.

1538 edition by Joannes Tacuinis de Cereto de Tridino. In Latin.

All other editions printed selections from the zoological and/or mineralogical sections. The last of these was that of 1552 by Herman Gülfferich at Frankfurt, a German translation.

◄§ 15 §►

Das Buch zu Distillieren of
Hieronymus Brunschwig

LTHOUGH the process of the distillation of liquids was well known before the end of the 15th century, and had been discussed in alchemical writings, Brunschwig's was the first major work to deal with it at length and in detail. The book, like Brunschwig himself, stood on the dividing line between the medieval and the modern world, for it was the last of the incunabula herbals and the first to be concerned with the chemistry and essential oils of plants. Brunschwig still drew upon the authorities of earlier ages, but many of his descriptions of medicinal plants and their uses were based on his own observations. In this sense he was more scientific than his predecessors.

In writing about his book it is difficult to know exactly which title to use. It is also difficult to determine what were the undisturbed contributions of Brunschwig himself, and what were additions or rearrangements made by his publisher, Grüninger. The book bears both a Latin title, *Liber de arte distillandi de Simplicibus,* and a German one, *Das distilier buch.* In addition, it exists in two versions, quite different in their content. One is called the *Kleine Destillierbuch,* the other the *Grosse Destillierbuch* (the small and the great book of distillation). Things are further complicated by the fact that the date of Brunschwig's death is unknown, so there is no way of knowing what edition was the last to receive his supervision. It has been suggested that he died in 1512, but that is also the year in which his *Grosse Destillierbuch* appeared for the first time.

Some of Brunschwig's statements reveal something of the man. For instance, we can assume that he had a more scientific mind than did many of his contemporaries, and that he valued accuracy. This emerges from his remarks about Grüninger's choice of illustrations. He advises the reader not to place too much reliance on the pictures, "for the figures are nothing more than a feast for the eyes, and for the information of those who cannot read or write." The cuts, indeed, are of little value, for they were borrowed from the repertoire that had been used for *Arbolayre,* the pirated editions of *Der Gart,* and the *Hortus sanitatis.*

Brunschwig, whose writings on distillation brought him lasting fame, was more of a surgeon than a physician. His first published writing was the *Cirurgia* of 1497. From hints in the text of that book we can gather that he was an army surgeon in 1475 and settled to practice at Strassburg in 1485. The *Cirurgia* was plagiarized by Schönsperger at Augsburg six months after its release, and this led to much of the bibliographic mixup that has plagued the Brunschwig works ever since. Grüninger, Brunschwig's Strassburg publisher, promptly inserted extra pages, reprinted others with corrections, added extra chapters, and so introduced a new edition to destroy the competition from Augsburg. Somewhat the same motive must have been behind the various states of *Das Distilierbuch.*

The *Cirurgia,* despite its title, is not concerned with the major operations then known, but with exterior wounds,

Das buch zu distillieren

die zusamen gethonen ding Compositि

ta genant/durch die eintzige ding/vnd das buch Thesaurus pau
perū/für die armen/durch experiment von mir Jheronymo
Brunschwick vff geklubt vnd geoffenbart/zū trost vñ
heil dē menschen vñ nutzlich ir leben vnd leib daruß
zū erlengeren vnd in gesuntheit zū behalten.

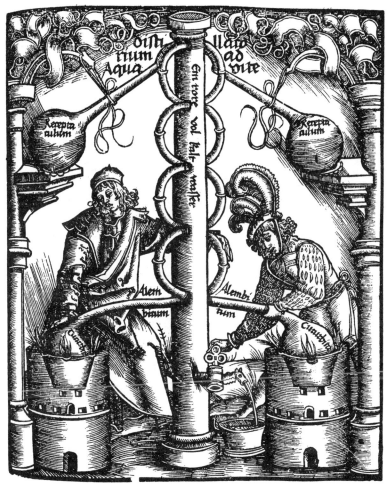

FIGURE 48. Title page of *Buch zu Distillieren*. The title page of Brunschwig's *Buch zu Distillieren* shows a rather fanciful apparatus. It looks more like something an alchemist might use than an apothecary's still. Nevertheless the basic principles involved are clearly shown. Vapors from a chosen substance are driven upward by heat and condensed into liquid. The liquid is collected, and then concentrated or refined still further. (From H. Brunschwig's *Das Buch zu Distillieren*. Strassburg, J. Grüninger, 1519. Original size 6″ wide × 9 1/4″ high.)

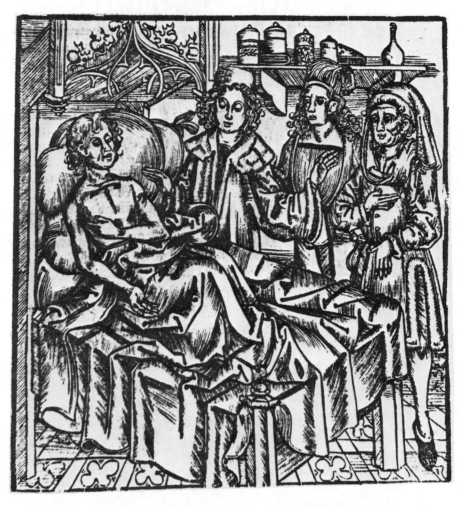

FIGURE 49. Sick-bed. Only a wealthy patient could afford the services of three physicians and the prescriptions they were apt to order. Medicine, if not altogether a perfected science in the early 16th century, was a profitable one, if the robes and furs of this trio of doctors are any indication. One of them even has a visibly full purse hanging from his belt. Perhaps they will prescribe potable gold, or crushed gemstones, and share in the apothecary's gains in addition to receiving their fees. (From Brunschwig's *Das Buch zu Distillieren*. Strassburg, J. Grüninger, 1519. Original size 5 ¹/₂" wide × 6 ⁵/₈" high.)

fractures, dislocations, and amputations. Its purpose was to aid "the surgeon living in lonely villages and castles far from all aid, who has to fall back on his own resources." That is a laudable intent, but one cannot help but wonder how the ultimate recipients of its advice, the wounded patients, fared from second-hand treatment.

The *Distilierbuch*, although it bore the Latin title *Liber de arte distillandi*, was written in German. It was through the vernacular that Brunschwig hoped to reach his intended audience, the general public, rather than merely the physicians and apothecaries. He devoted the entire first part of his book to the apparatus and methods of distillation, describing and showing the furnaces, stoves, retorts, alembics, pelicans, and other means of extracting and rectifying the juices of plants or those derived from animal products. Steam distillation, which preserves the essentials that would be destroyed by the direct heat of a fire, was the favored method. From distillation Brunschwig proceeded to a discussion of plants and their special attributes. The final section of his first edition gave an index of diseases along with remedies using distilled liquids. Distillation represented a positive advance over earlier therapy, because the active ingredients were generally made more effective through greater concentration and the drawing off of inert dross. It was an application of chemistry to the practice of medicine. Later and lengthier editions of the book increased the descriptive matter on apparatus, plants, and ailments. They also included sections on surgery and easily procured remedies, and an index to the errors made by the printer.

In Germany the *Distilierbuch* continued in print until after 1554. It was translated into English in 1527 and published in London at the Sygne of the Golden Crosse on Flete Strete. The publisher was Laurens Andrewe, who would later translate the Dutch *Der Dieren Pallys* (*The Palace of Animals*) into English about 1530. Quite possibly he performed the same service for Brunschwig using a copy brought back

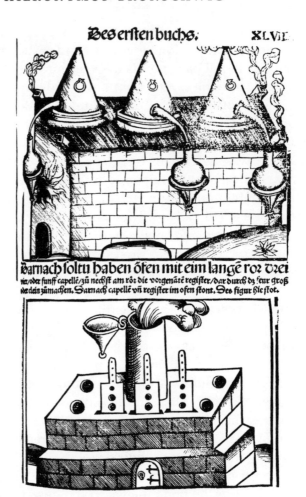

FIGURE 50. Stills and furnaces. The uppermost distiller's furnace, with its broad, flat top, permitted a number of vessels to be used at the same time. Draught was regulated by small vents in the corners, and heat was controlled simply by the amount and type of fuel. The lower furnace was somewhat more sophisticated. It had a stack that could be opened or closed, much like a damper, and graduated baffles that could increase or decrease air-flow above the firebox. (From Brunschwig's *Das Buch zu Distillieren*. Strassburg, J. Grüninger, 1519. Original size 5 7/16″ wide × 9 1/8″ high.)

from his long residence on the Continent, but this is uncertain since there is no mention of the translator's identity.

The English translation, which is of the *Kleine Destilierbuch*, is titled, in Tudor spelling, *"Ye Vertuose boke of Distillacyon of the waters of all maner of Herbes with the fygures of the styllatoryes fyrst made and compyled by the thyrte yeres study and labour of the moste connynge and famous Master of Phisycke Master Jherom Brunswyke."* In the preface are the following words, replete with the faith of the age: "Beholde how moche it excedeth to use medicyne of eficacye naturall by god ordeyned then wycked wordes or charmes of eficacie unnaturall by the devil envented."

No doubt Brunschwig's words were well heeded, for every manor house from the 15th century onward boasted of a still-room where herbal preparations were made and stored for future use. Through him the learning that originated in Salerno five centuries before filtered down to those who would otherwise have been without any kind of medical help. He termed himself "Hieronymus Brunschwyg, des geschlechts Salern, büntig von Strassburg," meaning that he was of the race of Salerno (i.e., a trained surgeon and physician) and validly of Strassburg. Brunfels referred to him as "nobilis," considering him to be of a noble German family, but again the facts elude us because Brunschwig was not specific. Had he said von Brunschwyg there would have been no doubt, but it would have been most unusual for one of noble birth to practice surgery, which was then usually done by barbers. In any case, through his humanitarian works, Brunschwig achieved nobility in the eyes of his fellow men.

BIBLIOGRAPHIC NOTES

1st edition: *Liber de arte distillandi de Simplicibus* (the *Kleines Destillierbuch*). 1500 by Johann Grüninger at Strassburg. Title in Latin but text in German. Many varying editions followed.

2nd major edition: (*Grosse Destillierbuch*). 1519 by Johann Grüninger at Strassburg.

Some editions contain three parts, others have five, but there are many other differences. For a full description of these see K. Sudhoff, in *Archiv fur Geschichte der Medizin* I, 1908, pages 41f, and 141f.

⤠ 16 ⤟

The *Herbarum Vivae Eicones* of Otto Brunfels

 H E modern age of botany began in 1530, when Otto Brunfels, a former theologian and monk, issued his *Herbarum vivae eicones* (*Living Images of Plants*). Within its covers we find some extremely realistic and beautiful plant pictures. Even by modern standards, they are of high quality. Of course some remarkably beautiful manuscript herbals had been produced earlier in Venice, all bearing skilfully painted pictures of herbs, trees, and flowers. But in regard to illustrations, none previously printed could equal the dazzling woodcuts presented in the *Herbarum vivae eicones.*

The artist responsible for the superb depictions was Hans von Weiditz, whose mastery has frequently been mistaken in the past for that of Dürer or of Burgkmair. Weiditz seems to have been the originator of most if not all of the designs, and appears to have supervised the draughtsmen and woodblock-cutters. This book was truly a case where the pictorial tail wagged the textual dog, as Brunfels lamented more than once. The order of the text followed that

in which the illustrations were completed, so any notion of a
botanical system perished before it was even born. Again
Brunfels had to be satisfied with depictions of some of the
local flora for which he had neither botanical names nor any
uses in medicine. Since the guilds of artists and artisans
more or less set the terms, it is most unlikely that Brunfels
himself was footing the bill for the illustrations. In all probability it was the printer-publisher Johann Schott who paid
for them. He certainly had a more than passing interest in
them, for the moment they were plagiarized he sued for re-
covery and was awarded the 132 cuts that had been copied
at considerable expense by Christian Egenolph of Frankfurt,
a rival publisher. Brunfels' part in the enterprise seems to
have been confined to providing the text as it was needed.
On one occasion he even apologized to the reader for having
included the picture of a plant that lacked a Latin name and
was unknown to medicine. That is scarcely the remark of a
man who had planned a scientifically useful herbal, and had
full control of its composition.

But in truth the innovative and progressive features of
Brunfels' herbal lie solely in the pictorial area. The plants
were keenly observed and drawn with a vigorous realism
that sometimes went beyond the needs of botany. If a plant
had a broken stem or a worm-eaten leaf, that was the way it
was shown. Except for an occasional excess, Weiditz had a
superb grasp of plant structure.

FIGURE 51. Title page of Brunfels' herbal. The title page of Brunfels' *Herbarum Vivae Eicones* is richly allegorical in content, as are those of many
other 16th- and 17th-century books. Hercules subduing the dragon who
guarded the Golden Apples of the Hesperides is an obvious allusion to
the life-restoring gifts of medicine. The physician, Dioscorides, and
Apollo, god of the arts and sciences, are also understandable elements,
while Venus and Silenus probably represent two of the most frequent
causes for calling on the physician's services. (From Brunfels' *Herbarum
Vivae Eicones*. Strassburg, J. Schott, 1530. Original size 6 $7/16$" wide ×
9 $11/16$" high.)

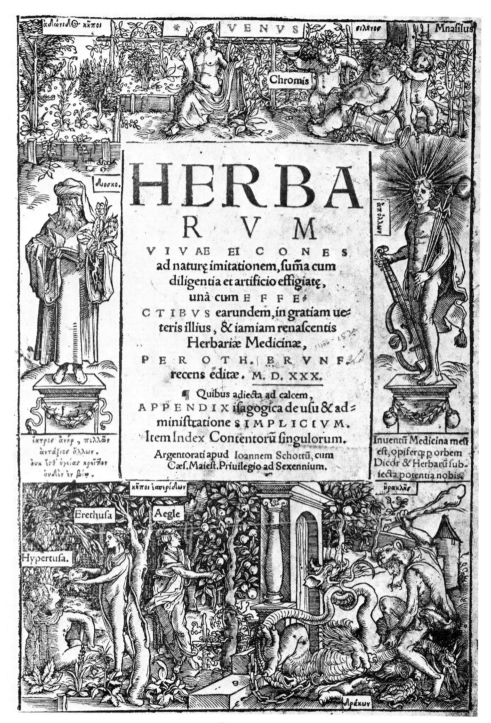

HERBA
RVM

VIVAE EICONES
ad naturę imitationem, suma cum
diligentia et artificio effigiatę,
unà cum EFFE:
CTIBVS earundem, in gratiam ue:
teris illius, & iamiam renascentis
Herbariæ Medicinæ,
PER OTH. BRVNF.
recens editæ. M. D. XXX.

¶ Quibus adiecta ad calcem,
APPENDIX isagogica de usu & ad:
ministratione SIMPLICIVM.
Item Index Contentorũ singulorum.

Argentorati apud Ioannem Schottũ, cum
Cæs. Maiest. Priuilegio ad Sexennium.

FIGURE 51.

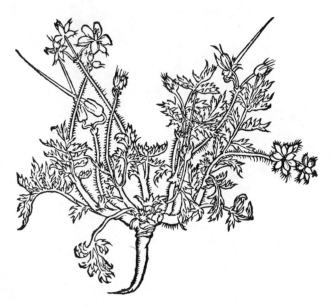

FIGURE 52. Geranium. Herb Robert was known to Brunfels as Storken-schnabel or Crane's Bill, and to us as Geranium. It was used in treating kidney-stones, to stanch blood, and most particularly to heal cuts and wounds. Its styptic and astringent qualities were called upon in cases of internal bleeding and hemorrhoids, as well as for healing old ruptures. It was taken internally, usually with wine, or externally as an application. The beaklike seed pods are responsible for the name Crane's Bill. (From Brunfels' *Herbarum Vivae Eicones*. Strassburg, J. Schott, 1530. Original size 4 1/8" wide × 4 3/16" high.)

Some of Weiditz's watercolors for the woodcuts were discovered during the early 1930s in the Felix Platter Herbarium at Berne. Quite understandably they outshine the woodcuts based upon them, for they have the advantage of modelled coloration, while the prints that evolved from them were limited to pure line. Weiditz, in the watercolors, showed an understanding of botanical needs that was somewhat ahead of his time. He surrounded some of the plants with separate details picturing leaves, petals, seeds, and other identifying features essential to the botanist.

Ever since Julius Sachs, an historian of botany, first coined the phrase, "the German fathers of botany," Brunfels

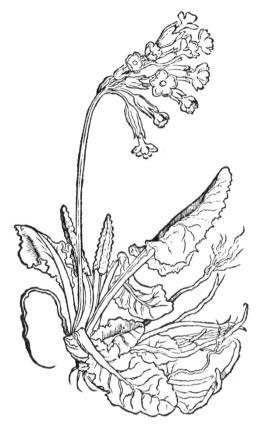

FIGURE 53. Herba Paralysis. The ordinary cowslip or primrose was known by several other names: paigle, St. Peter's keys, Heaven's keys, and Herba Paralysis. The fancied resemblance to a bunch of keys easily explains two of the terms, but for the reference to paralysis it is necessary to go back to Greek medicine, which prescribed it for palsies, paralytic ailments, and rheumatisms, since it had a sedative and antispasmodic action. (From Brunfels' *Herbarum Vivae Eicones*. Strassburg, J. Schott, 1530. Original Size 3 ³/₁₆″ wide × 6 ³/₁₆″ high.)

has been considered to be the pioneer of the group. But a closer look at Brunfels' work dispels some of that aura of majesty. To begin with, there are no true botanical descriptions in *Herbarum vivae eicones*, and there are occasions

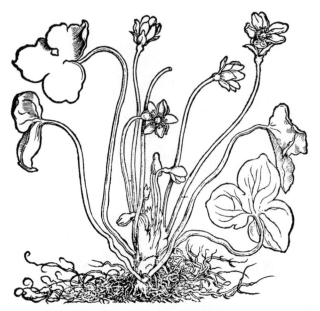

FIGURE 54. Hepatica. As its very name implies, Hepatica was considered an excellent remedy for liver ailments, especially jaundice, and was also used to heal sores, scabs, and the bites of mad dogs. In the latter case the patient was bled of ten ounces on each of four successive days, before drinking powdered liverwort and pepper in warm milk. That was followed by two or three sea baths daily for a month, with long immersion periods (the longer the better) being recommended. (From Brunfels' *Herbarum Vivae Eicones*. Strassburg, J. Schott, 1530. Original size 4 1/2" wide × 5 1/8" high.)

when the pictures do not correspond to the text. It seems almost as if Brunfels did not proof the pages, and left that task to the publisher. On matters pertaining to botany Brunfels was woefully lacking. His text draws upon all the earlier authorities of the medieval, Arabic, and classical eras, and his main intention was to establish a harmony or concordance between the flora of transalpine Germany and that presented by Greek and Arabic authors. Theophrastus had been aware, some 2,000 years earlier, that species differed from place to place, and that the flora of one region was not the same as that of another. Brunfels remained unaware of

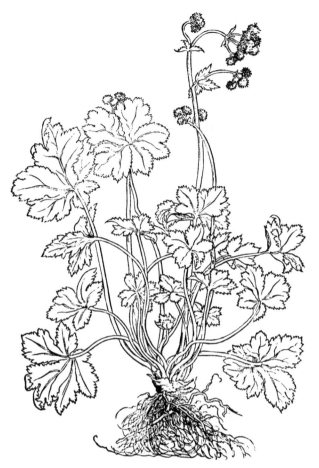

FIGURE 55. Sanicle (All Heal). This herb grows in shaded woodland throughout almost all of Europe. Its astringent and styptic qualities gained for it a great reputation for healing wounds, probably a result of its tannin content. It belongs in the same order as the mints, the Labiatae, and was anciently known as Prunella and Brunella. When it migrated to America it gained two other names: Blue Curls and Heart of the Earth. (From Brunfels' *Herbarum Vivae Eicones.* Strassburg, J. Schott, 1530. Original size 6″ wide × 9 ⁹⁄₁₆″ high.)

that elementary fact, but was not unique in so erring. Botany, at that time, still lacked the data and methods which we take for granted today.

At every turn it is more apparent that Brunfels' knowledge of botany was obtained from books rather than nature. As a physician he had to know something about the herbs that were used to treat particular ailments, but it is doubtful that he gathered his own stock of medicinal plants. After all, that was a function of the apothecary, so there was no need for one who used plant materials in prescription to be able to recognize the growing plant in nature. Much of what Brunfels gathered about plants came from herbalist friends, such as Hieronymous Bock, and from the lore of old country wives and herb-women. Some of his information was practical, some pure fantasy (such as the notion that masculine plants were of a deeper color, stronger in action, and better formed than the so-called feminine ones). None of this information, however, was original with Brunfels.

If, perhaps, he has been wrongly credited in areas where he was not deserving, there are others where high praise is clearly due him. Brunfels as a botanist is one thing, as a human being quite another. Bock's Herbal, with its highly descriptive text and regard for ecology and plant communities, was encouraged by Brunfels, who insisted that Bock write it for the benefit of his countrymen. Brunfels, in fact, walked forty miles just to speak to him about it.

Brunfels had a sense of dedication through his rather brief life that seems to have grown out of genuine religious conviction. The son of a cooper, he was born c. 1489 in the town of Braunfels, near Mainz. He was educated at Mainz, where he took a masters degree around 1510. Somewhat later, Brunfels entered a Carthusian monastery, where he remained until he was caught up in the fever of the Reformation. He fled the monastery in 1521, and for a time became an itinerant Lutheran preacher through southern Germany. In 1524 he settled in Strassburg, opened a small school, and married. During the succeeding years he devoted himself to theology, botany, and medicine, finally publishing the *Herbarum vivae eicones* in 1530. Also in 1530 he took a degree in medicine at the University of Basel, and in 1532 was appointed Town Physician of Berne. His good fortune, however, was short-lived. He died in 1534, at the age of 45. Although not a "father of botany," he did make two genuine and lasting contributions to his beloved science. One was the arena for Weiditz's art; the other was the inspiration for the first "scientific" herbal, that of Hieronymous Bock.

BIBLIOGRAPHIC NOTES

1st edition: 1530 by Johann Schott at Strassburg. The work was issued in three parts: Part 1 in 1530, Part 2 in 1532, and Part 3 in 1536. In Latin.

A German translation appeared in 1532 under the title *Contrafayt Kreüterbuch* in folio size. The second part, called *Ander Teyl des Teütsch en Contrafayten Kreüterbuchs*, appeared in 1537, also folio size.

A quarto edition, using the cuts recovered from Christian Egenolph of Frankfurt, was published in 1534, under the title *Kreüterbuch Contrafayt*.

2nd edition of the Latin *Herbarum vivae eicones* was published in three parts: Part 1 in 1532, Part 2 in 1536, and Part 3 in 1540.

3rd edition of the Latin version appeared as *Herbarium Othonis Brunfelsii tomis tribus*. Part 1 is dated 1539, but the book contains the parts 2 and 3 used in the 1536 and 1540 issuances of the 2nd edition.

All editions above by Johann Schott at Strassburg.

All illustrated by Hans von Weiditz, save Part 3 of all editions, for which other artists, among them Master I. K., were used.

The *Kreüter Buch* of Hieronymus Bock

HILE Brunfels is commonly given the credit for initiating the modern era in botany, that honor properly belongs to Hieronymus Bock. On the title page of his herbal, Bock set forth his limited but highly consequential purpose: to discuss the characteristics, effects, and names of the plants that grew in Germany. This meant considerably more than is apparent at first glance. It meant that Bock had taken a totally different direction from that represented by the traditional medico-botanical works of his day. The business of identifying the plants of Dioscorides, heretofore the prime concern of physicians, herbalists, and botanists, was now relegated to a secondary place. It also meant that, since Bock wrote about German plants, his qualifications and material came from his own surroundings and experience, and were not derived from the opinions and observations of others.

Those factors by themselves would not have made his work unique, but to them he added yet another idea: the notion of a *system* of botany. As Theophrastus had done al-

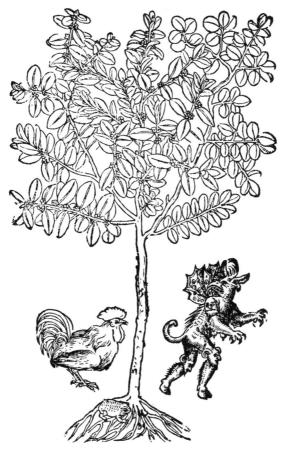

FIGURE 56. Buxbaum. In many parts of Europe, particularly in the north where not many plants were apt to be in leaf by Palm Sunday, box became a substitute for palm. The association of the plant with Christ's entry into Jerusalem thus came into being, and that connection with the Easter story is why the Devil is shown running from it in terror at cockcrow. (From Bock's *Kreuter Buch*. Strassburg, W. Rihel, 1546. Original size 3 ⁵/₈" wide × 6 ¹/₁₆" high.)

most 2,000 years earlier, Bock put plants into three broad classifications; herbs, shrubs, and trees. But he did more than that. Within those extensive groups, he arranged plants into categories based on similar appearance, qualities, or other indications of relationship. The arrangement was neither accidental nor borrowed from the investigations of others, but resulted from Bock's recognition that the prevalent alphabetical systems of arranging plants introduced both error and disparity. Bock did not introduce the concepts of genus and species, but his work paved the way for their development by such later botanists as Cesalpino, Bauhin, and the famed Linnaeus.

Bock, who was born in 1498 at Heidelsheim near Bretten, had been intended for the monastery by his parents, but a cloistered life was not for him. He went to the university instead, where he studied medicine, and he later became a schoolteacher at Zweibrucken in the Palatinate region, about 50 miles northwest of Strassburg. From 1523 to 1532 he was superintendent of the gardens of the Count Palatine Ludwig. No doubt the bulk of his highly practical botanical education was gained there. Following the death of his patron, Bock became pastor of a Lutheran church at nearby Hornbach, but was driven away by the effects of the Counter Reformation. He returned to that post after a period of privation, and remained there until his death in 1554. His dual career, incidentally, was not unique, for throughout the 16th century there were a great number of Protestant clergymen who were also engaged in botanical pursuits.

Lacking the money to have his herbal properly illustrated, Bock hit upon another idea that was to be of great value to the future of botany. He wrote in such a clear and detailed manner that even a layman could determine what plants he was talking about. He thus created the prototype of modern phytography, the science of plant description. Bock's writing is not filled with complicated terminology. The material is presented in a simple, vivid, even racy style that went straight to the point and troubled itself very little with Dioscorides, the Arabic physicians, or other pundits of the past. There is also a good deal on plant communities and

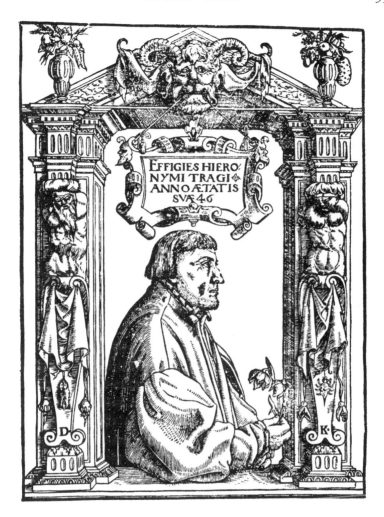

FIGURE 57. Portrait of Bock. David Kandel, a young artist chosen to illustrate Bock's *Kreutter Buch* in its second edition, gave us this depiction of Jerome Bock at age 46. Despite Bock's aversion to the lustfully goatish and sinful implications of his name (Bock meaning he-goat in German) Kandel has figured a satyr's mask with resplendent goat-horns directly above the inscription and portrait. Translating his name into the Latin (Tragus) seems to have done the author very little good. (From Bock's *Kreuter Buch*. Strassburg, W. Rihel, 1546. Original size 4 9/16″ wide × 6 1/4″ high.)

plant environment. In a sense, Bock was a 16th-century eco-
logist.

Despite its genuine and laudable scientific contributions, the *Kreüter Buch* of 1539 needed pictorial help to be of
greatest value to its audience. About seven years went by,
however, before young David Kandel, a self-taught illustrator, provided some 365 woodcuts for the second edition, in
1546. Many of them were copied from the cuts in Brunfels'
Herbarum vivae eicones and Fuchs's *Historia stirpium*. But the
genre scenes, which give a unique flavor to Bock's herbal,
and are a kind of visual counterpart to the prose, were original with Kandel. He even provided a portrait of Bock, seen
in profile, which must have been done in 1544, for it reads
"at his age 46." The decorative border surrounding it is
quite accomplished, but it contains one element that may
not have been entirely to Bock's liking. That is the satyr's
head that crowns the frame and sports a magnificent set of
goat's horns. Bock's surname in German meant he-goat, and
he was quite sensitive about it, for it bore connotations in
his native language that were most inappropriate to a
clergyman. The he-goat was a symbol of Satan, and was also
an attribute of one of the Seven Deadly Sins, Lust, often
depicted riding on the back of a he-goat. For that reason
Bock Latinized his name to Tragus, hoping to make it less
recognizable.

It seems unlikely that Bock was well versed in Latin,
however, for when his publisher wished to issue a Latin
edition, he engaged a young scholar named David Kyber to
translate the Bavarian dialect of Bock. Kyber finished the
task in 1552, just one year before he was fatally stricken by
the plague at the age of 28.

Of a piece with Bock's practicality and his desire to
speak in understandable language was his rejection of superstition and misinformation. Dioscorides had said fern
produced no seed, while the German peasants said it did.
They, however, surrounded its production and gathering

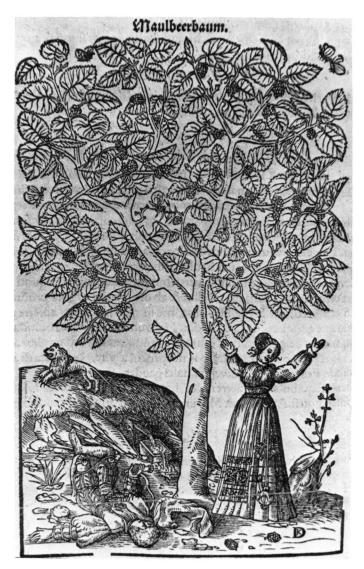

FIGURE 58. Mulberry; Pyramus and Thisbe. Kandel gave vent to his story-telling leanings from time to time, in this case by including the tale of Pyramus and Thisbe played out beneath the branches of a mulberry tree. The lion fleeing in the background, after dining on an ox, was responsible for Pyramus believing Thisbe to have been killed. He promptly killed himself beneath a mulberry tree, which became stained ever after with his blood, hence the red mulberry. (From Bock's *Kreutterbuch*. Strassburg, W. Rihel, 1556. Original size 3 $^{11}/_{16}$" wide × 6 $^{1}/_{8}$" high.)

with all manner of supernatural hazards. Bock settled the matter to his own satisfaction by investigating the plant on four successive Midsummer Eves, when fern seed was said to be formed. He simply set sheets and mullein leaves beneath fronds of bracken, thereby catching the spores without the use of charms, spells, or other forms of witchcraft and, quite incidentally, proving himself a better botanist than Dioscorides and the other ancients. Bock was an amateur botanist, largely self-taught and completely self-reliant, but his accomplishments moved the study of plants closer to a science of botany than any individual had done since Theophrastus wrote his *Enquiry into Plants* in the 4th century B.C.

BIBLIOGRAPHIC NOTES

1st edition: 1539 by Wendel Rihel at Strassburg. No illustrations.

2nd edition: 1546 by Wendel Rihel at Strassburg. Illustrations by David Kandel.

3rd edition: 1551 by Wendel Rihel at Strassburg. In the years 1553, 1556, 1560, 1565, 1572, and 1574 the *Kreüter Buch* was issued at Strassburg by Josias Rihel. Five more editions under the editorship of Melchior Sebizius appeared in 1577, 1580, 1586, 1587, and 1595 at Strassburg.

A Latin translation by David Kyber was printed in 1552 by Wendel Rihel at Strassburg.

A picture-book edition with plant names and short descriptions was published in 1553 by Wendel Rihel at Strassburg.

All the editions after the first of 1539 carried the David Kandel woodcuts.

❧ 18 ☙

The *De Historia Stirpium* of Leonhart Fuchs

UCHS, like Brunfels before him, was largely concerned with bringing about much-needed reforms in German medicine and pharmacy. His dedicatory letter in *De historia stirpium* complained that hardly one doctor in a hundred had knowledge of so much as a handful of plants. Doctors counted on the largely illiterate apothecaries who, in turn, relied on the old peasants who gathered roots and herbs. Fuchs was keenly aware that this careless procedure not only caused errors but was dangerous. A patient could very easily be poisoned rather than cured through improper identification of plant material.

Since the materia medica of the 16th century was still based on the classical authorities, it was only natural that Fuchs sought to provide his readers with the plant descriptions of Dioscorides, Pliny, and Galen. To this text he added clearly delineated figures of the plants themselves, so that there could be no error or equivocation. Brunfels, as Fuchs had noted, had run into occasional difficulties when it came

137

to matching pictures with text, and Fuchs took great care
that such mistakes would not occur in his book. The plants
were arranged in the order of the Greek alphabet, which
Fuchs hoped would be a convenience. Four indices were
supplied: the first in Greek, the second in Latin, a third
which gave the apothecaries' and herbalists' names for the
plants, and the fourth in German. But it is not always easy
to determine where to find what, since the *chapter* headings
are in Greek and the plant figures accompanying them are
labelled in Latin and German. This is not too difficult with
something like Maiden-hair, which is *Adiantos* in Greek,
Adiantum in Latin, and *Frawenhar* in German. But when you
have *Acalyphe* in the Greek, *Urtica romana* in Latin, and
Welschnessel in German, things become somewhat un-
wieldy. Another trap for the unwary modern is Fuchs's use
of the terms "masculine" and "feminine." These words in
no sense mean that Fuchs recognized plants to have sexual
characteristics. Rather, it was a convenient (?) means of dis-
tinguishing related species on the basis of stronger or
weaker qualities.

The *Historia stirpium* was a learned work for its day, and
reflected the careful scholarship of its author. Fuchs was
born at Wemding in Bavaria in the year 1501. He matricu-
lated at the University of Erfurt in 1513, and distinguished
himself there in Greek and Latin studies. In 1519 he went to
Ingolstadt, where he took a doctorate in 1524. Shortly thereafter he began medical practice in Munich. Then, in quick
succession, he taught medicine at Ingolstadt in 1526, became
court-physician to the Margrave Georg von Brandenburg in
1528, and returned to Ingolstadt in 1533 as professor. Having
become a Lutheran, he left the Catholic town of Ingolstadt in
1535 to become professor of medicine at the new Protestant
University of Tübingen. There he remained until his death
in 1566. During a year when there was an outbreak of sweating sickness, Fuchs provided a successful treatment. As a
result his fame spread abroad and he was offered foreign

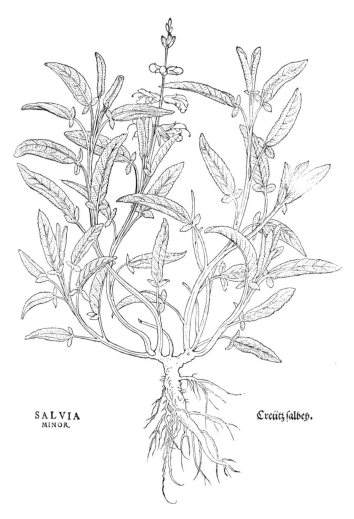

SALVIA
MINOR.

Creütz falbey.

FIGURE 59. Salvia (Sage). Sage was in high repute as a medicament from ancient times. Indeed, there was a traditional saying, "Why should a man die whilst sage grows in his garden?" Once it was even traded in China by the Dutch merchants, who cannily obtained three ounces of the finest tea leaves for every ounce of sage. Now used almost entirely as a condiment, sage was once used for almost everything from snake bite to the plague. (From Fuchs's *De Historia Stirpium*. Basle, M. Isingrin, 1542. Reduced from original size, 7 ¹/₂" wide × 10 ³/₄" high.)

LEONHARTVS FVCH-
SIVS, AETATIS SVAE
ANNO XLI.

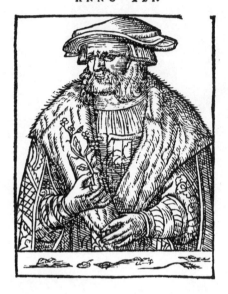

FIGURE 60. Small portrait of Fuchs. This portrait, showing Leonart Fuchs at age 41, is from the 1549 edition by B. Arnolletum of Lyon. It is a reduced and reversed version of the one that appeared as a full-length figure in the Basle edition of 1542. The French edition, while lacking the grand scale of the original, did have the virtue of portability, since it could be carried about in the rather voluminous costumes of the time. It was, in a sense, among the early examples of a field guide. (From Fuchs's *De Historia Stirpium*. Lyon, B. Arnolletum, 1549 12 mo. ed. Original size 1 7/8" wide × 2 1/2" high.)

posts, all of which he declined. Although the first editions of *De historia stirpium* were financial failures, his great reputation insured a large and continuing sale for later printings. Many, however, brought nothing to Fuchs since they were produced in France and elsewhere.

The truly important thing about Fuchs's herbal is not his text, scholarly as it may be, but rather the illustrations

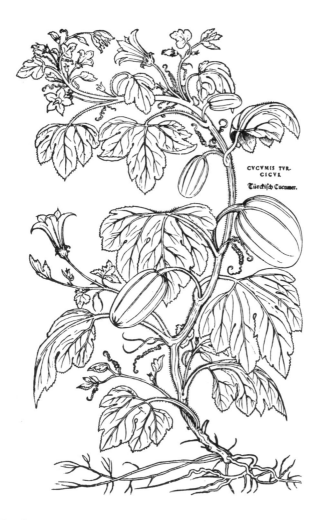

FIGURE 61. *Cucumis turcicus.* The Vegetable Marrow was not a Turkish Cucumber, despite Fuchs's designation of it as such. Its scientific name is *Cucurbita pepo,* and, since it belongs to the very confusing and variable family of the *Cucurbitaceae,* it is related to that Halloween and Thanksgiving treat, the pumpkin. The seeds of this plant were an effective vermifuge, but for mechanical rather than chemical reasons. (From Fuchs's *De Historia Stirpium.* Basle, M. Isingrin, 1542. Reduced from original size, 8" wide × 13" high.)

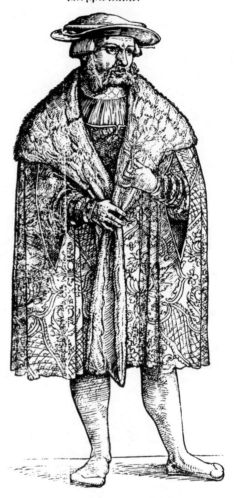

FIGURE 62. Full-length portrait of Fuchs. Dr. Leonhart Fuchs as he appeared in 1542, when he was a
full professor at the University of Tubingen and had
completed his famous *De Historia Stirpium*. This
print from it bears an erroneous age, for he was
only 42 when the same print was published in Den
Nieuwen Herbarius of 1543, a Low German version
of Fuchs's herbal issued by Isingrin of Basle, who
certainly knew that his author had not aged seven
years in the space of one. (From Fuchs's *Den Nieuwen Herbarius*. Basle, M. Isingrin, 1543. Original
size 4 $^1/_2$″ wide × 10 $^1/_{16}$″ high.)

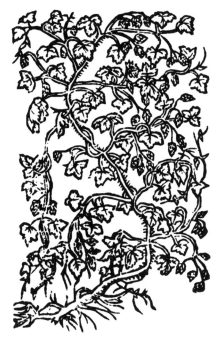

FIGURE 63. Lupulus (Hops). Hops (*Humulus lupulus*) have long been known to have other uses than flavoring ale and beer. The dried flower heads or cones, called strobiles, possess a volatile oil that induces a calming effect and brings on sleep when the scent is inhaled. Fibers from the plant have also been used to manufacture a coarse, woven cloth, and paper has been made from the stems. (From Fuchs's *De Historia Stirpium*. Lyon, B. Arnolletum, 1549. Original size 1 1/2" wide × 3" high.)

that he obtained for it. They were done under the close supervision of Fuchs himself, who saw to it that the designers and engravers adhered to a plan and did not exceed certain limits, as they had with Brunfels. There are some who praise Fuchs's herbal as the most artistic of all, but there are others who claim that Brunfels' *Herbarum* is superior. In Fuchs's work the line is lighter in character, almost too light for the scale of a full folio page, but there is almost always a sensitive handling of design, and certainly greater

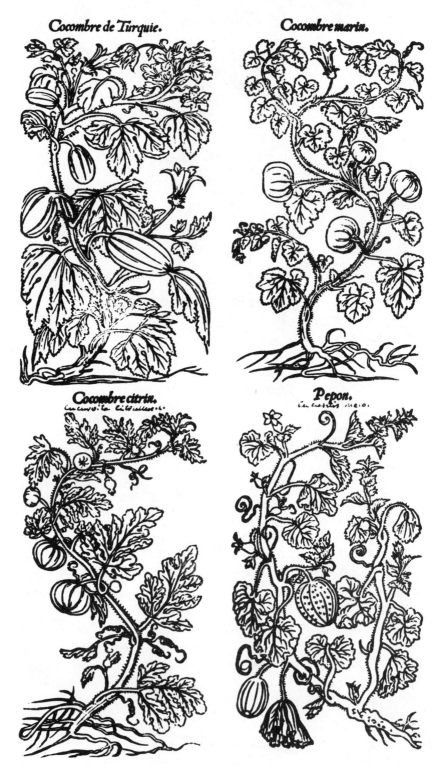

Cocombre de Turquie.

Cocombre marin.

Cocombre citrin.

Pepon.

FIGURE 64.

stress on botanical necessities. William Morris, John Ruskin, and Agnes Arber, all well qualified to judge, thought highly enough of the work to purchase first folio editions. There is a sizable school of opinion, however, that prefers the reduced cuts which illustrate the octavo size editions, for there the lines seem to have gained in vigor and to have lost any hint of objectionable thinness.

The artists that Fuchs chose to do his illustrations were the best available in Basel, and their skill is evident in the 509 cuts that they created. Fuchs singled them out for praise, and included their portraits in the *Historia stirpium.* Heinrich Füllmaurer is seen transferring the designs to the woodblocks and Albrecht Mayer is shown preparing the drawings, while Veit Rudolph Speckle, the master cutter, sits in solitary splendor in the register just below them. Clearly the era of the anonymous artist, author, and craftsman was over.

One of the illustrations included in the *Historia* was the first representation of maize, our familiar corn. Fuchs was misinformed of its origin, however, for he calls it Turkish rather than American. In describing it, his text refers to four colors—yellow, reddish purple, red, and white—as the characteristic colors of corn, and they are shown in that sequence in the illustrations of the surviving colored copies. A picture of a plum tree is divided into three zones—yellow at the left, blue in the center, and pinkish-red on the right to represent three kinds of plum trees. A depiction of *Lamium* shows shoots of yellow, mauve, and white, always in that order, while a picture of roses is white on the left side and

FIGURE 64. Four cucurbits. Later editions of Fuchs's herbal carried reduced versions of the large folio-size pictures used in the edition of 1542. Four of the smaller cuts took up only about half the space demanded by the originals. These cucurbits have lost little or no necessary detail in the process of being cut down, as may be noted by comparing the smaller Vegetable Marrow with its larger parent. (From Fuchs's *Commentaires tres excellens de l'hystoire des plantes.* Paris, 1549. Original size 5 5/8" wide × 10 1/8" high.)

red on the right. The consistency of the coloring from copy to copy would seem to indicate that the books were issued with coloring, rather than being colored later by individual owners. It is known that the Plantin establishment at Antwerp had a small staff of colorists, and that the Brunfels herbal (when colored) was colored by skilful hands. Unfortunately the coloring in the Fuchs herbal is not of a high quality, often hiding graceful outlines behind an opaque wash of pigment. It does, however, give evidence that the hand-colored illustration was an early feature of the book trade.

It should be noted that the *Historia stirpium* has other merits in addition to its woodcuts: in it are the descriptions of more than a hundred plants never before mentioned; it provides a record of the plants introduced into 16th century Germany from elsewhere; and some of the figures became the "historic types" referred to by Linnaeus in his monumental system of classification. But these elements have greater significance for the botanist than for the layman, so that, in the final analysis, it is the illustrations that are of greatest value. They formed the basis for an entire series of pictures used to illustrate the works of Turner and Dodoens, and they were also adapted by David Kandel for use in Bock's *Kreüter Buch*.

BIBLIOGRAPHIC NOTES

1st edition: 1542 by Michael Isingrin at Basel, under the title *De historia stirpium*. Folio size.

2nd edition: 1543 by Michael Isingrin at Basel. German translation and revision of the *Historia*, now titled *New Kreüterbuch*. Folio size.

3rd edition: 1545 by Isingrin at Basel. This was with plant names only, no text, and the illustrations were newly cut to a reduced size. Title was *Läbliche Abbildung und Contrafaytung aller Kreüter . . .* Octavo size.

4th edition: same date, printer, and place. Title was *Primi de stirpium historia commentariorum tomi vivae Imagines.* Latin names, but no text. Octavo size.

5th edition: same date, printer, and place. Dutch translation titled *Den Nieuwen Herbarius.* Folio size. This was the last edition directly under Isingrin's control, for he sold the cuts to the Parisian printer Gazeau. For further information on the subsequent editions see Stübler's monograph, *Leonhart Fuchs,* published 1928.

Isingrin's printer's device was a cast type capital letter I resting in the branches of a shrub, thus forming a rebus (I is in green).

The octavo and duodecimo editions, especially the octavo without text by Balthasar Arnoullet (Lyons, 1549), are fine examples in convenient size of the Fuchs illustrations. They are, in fact, 16th-century fieldguides.

The *New Herball* of William Turner

NGLISH botany can properly be said to begin with the herbal of William Turner, a work that suffered as many vicissitudes as did its author during the seventeen years it took to complete. Prior to Turner the only books in English even remotely connected with botany were Banckes's *Herbal* of 1525, and *The Grete Herball* of 1526. Both were thoroughly medieval in character, and were based on European plants rather than English ones. The state of plant knowledge in England in Turner's time was dismal, to say the least, as the following quote will make clear. While at Cambridge, Turner complained that "I could learne never one Greke, nether Latin nor English name, even amongest the Phisiciones, of any herbe or tre, such was the ignorance in simples at that tyme."

One of the first steps he took to rectify that situation was the publication of his *Libellus de re herbaria novus* (*The New Little Book About Plants*) in the year 1538. Ten years later he issued *The Names of Herbes in Greke, Latin, Englishe,*

Duche and Frenche Wyth the Commune Names That Herbaries and Apotecaries Use, thus providing a wealth of new and useful information for English readers.

Turner was born in Morpeth, Northumberland, near the beginning of the 16th century. He must have impressed his schoolmasters favorably, for he was sent to Cambridge University, Pembroke College, at the expense of Lord Wentworth. Turner was elected a Fellow of the College in 1530, after receiving his Baccalaureate. He began his Master's degree in 1533. In 1538 he was senior treasurer, the same year he published the *Libellus*. The work made mention of many Northumberland plants that had never before been described. But along with his botanical information he included some remarks on a more controversial subject, theology and the Reformation. His mentor at Cambridge, Nicholas Ridley, had taught him Greek, tennis, archery, and also the art of being a Nonconformist, which meant that he refused to accept the dictates of the Church of England. This had unfortunate consequences, particularly when Turner left Cambridge to preach his views throughout England. It happened to be the England of Henry VIII, so Turner went to jail for two years, was exiled to the Continent on his release, and saw the destruction of all his published works.

Turner put his banishment to good use, however, and learned from the leading scientists of Europe, men such as Conrad Gesner and Luca Ghini. He even took a Doctorate in Medicine, at either Ferrara or Bologna, and spent much of his time botanizing through Italy, Switzerland, Germany, and Holland. No doubt he was gathering material for his herbal throughout those wanderings while waiting for the chance to return home. When Henry died, the way was opened for the exile to return as a loyal subject of Edward VI. In short order Turner was appointed physician and chaplain to the Lord Protector Edward Duke of Somerset, and was made Prebendary of York and Dean of Wells, since he was a divine as much as he was a doctor or botanist.

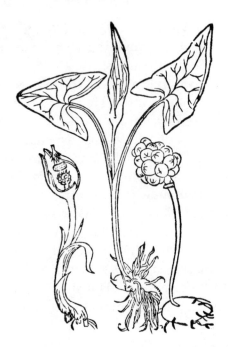

FIGURE 65. Cuckoo pynt. *Arum maculatum*, which Turner called Cuckoo-pint, is also known as Lords and Ladies, Rampe, and Wake Robin, the last from its habit of blooming when the robins arrived. Its powdered root was used cosmetically to bleach freckles, and the fresh tubers were stewed with lard to make an ointment for ringworm. Starch from its tuberous roots once stiffened Elizabethan ruffs. (From William Turner's *A New Herball*. Collen, A. Birckman, 1568. Original size 2 ⁵/₈″ wide × 5 ¹/₈″ high.)

During Edward's brief six-year reign Turner managed to finish the first part of his herbal. He published it in London in 1551, and dedicated it to the Duke of Somerset. But with the death of Edward everything reverted to its former disastrous state. Mary I, a Catholic Queen with little taste for the Reformation, came to the throne. For the second time Turner's books were banned, and this time his herbal was included as well. Complete copies of the first part of Turner's

Of Anagyris.

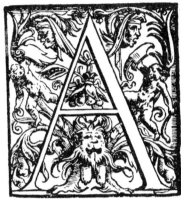

Anagyris groweth not in Englande that I wote of/but I haue sene it in Italye. It may be called in English Beane trifolye/becaufe the leaues growe thre together/and the sede is muche lyke a Beane. Anagyris is a bushe lyke vnto a tree with leues and twigges/like vnto Agnus castus of Italy. But the leaues are greater and shorter/and growe but thre together/where as Agnus hath euer fyue together/and excedinge stinkinge/wherevpon riseth the Prouerb/Præstat hanc Anagyrim nō attigifle. It hath the floures lyke vnto kole. It hath a fruyt in longe horned coddes/of the lykenes of a kidney/of diuerfe coloures/firme and stronge/whiche when the grape is ripe wexeth harde.

FIGURE 66. Anagyris (text and decorative initial). Seeds of Anagyris, as Turner said, would indeed "maketh one vomite sore," for they contained an alkaloid (Cytisine) which is also found in the poisonous Laburnum. Aside from external use Anagyris was a dangerous remedy that could cause coma, convulsions, and severe diarrhea. Minute amounts were used to treat asthma and whooping cough, and perhaps the creature under the bar of the letter A has just had a dose of it. (From William Turner's *A New Herball*. Collen, A. Birckman, 1568. Original size 5 $^{3}/_{8}$″ wide × 3 $^{3}/_{8}$″ high.)

New Herball are almost never met with, since most of them were sought out and destroyed.

There followed a second period of exile during which Turner continued his examination of European plants while preparing the second part of his work. It took five years, however, before he could return to England and be restored to favor by Elizabeth I, thus regaining all of his posts. At one of their meetings the Queen conversed with him in Latin. She apparently held him in high regard, for on four separate occasions Elizabeth granted her contentious subject the great seal of England to insure his protection. Rarely, if ever, had a botanist required so much protection from the state, but then few botanists had become so involved in religious disputes and high politics.

In his religious role he was completely intractable, proclaiming from the pulpit the most extreme views. He would have nothing whatever to do with religious ceremony. He even taught his dog to snatch away bishops' caps on a given signal. In 1564 Elizabeth regretfully saw Turner forced to retire to his home in London.

His retirement came two years after the second part of the *New Herball* appeared (in 1562) from the press of Arnold Birckman of Cologne. Turner apparently chose a foreign publisher because he didn't trust the continued freedom of the English press. Besides, Birckman had access to the Fuchs series of woodcuts, which he wanted for illustrations.

In his crowded quarters at Crutched Friars, Turner doggedly proceeded with part three of his herbal and finished it only a few months before his death in 1568. Quite fittingly it is dedicated to Elizabeth, who saw to it that all things English stayed English and free, including thorny botanists with a penchant for making enemies. The third part, incidentally, was bound together with the first and second parts. The parts had been revised, rewritten, corrected, and enlarged, thus forming what amounted to a new work, and the only complete edition of Turner's herbal.

Over 200 species native to England are described in Turner's pages, and some of them were first named by him. Like other physicians of his time, Turner was concerned with the proper identification of the medicinal materials of Dioscorides, but he was by no means overawed by his predecessor's authority, and differed with him on more than one occasion. Turner was well aware that the local northern floras did not agree with those written about by Dioscorides, Galen, and Pliny, and that the British flora was often distinct from the Continental floras. He also scoffed at

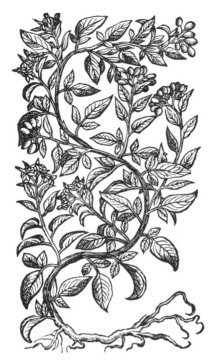

FIGURE 67. Bittersweet. Amaradulcis or Bittersweet is one of the Solanaceae, *Solanum dulcamara*. It is one of the most common plants found in hedgerows and along ditches, and is often mistaken for Belladonna. Shepherds once used it to protect their sheep from the evil eye, but Linnaeus recommended it for rheumatism, fever, and inflammatory diseases. Today it is employed for obstinate skin eruptions and chronic bronchial catarrh. (From William Turner's *A New Herball*. Collen, A. Birckman, 1568. Original size 2 9/16" wide × 5 1/2" high.)

many of the old superstitions, such as the belief that the mandrake root had a human form. He cautioned against overuse of any herb, being a moderate as a doctor if not as a divine, and offered a most unusual remedy for an overdose of opium: "if the pacient be to much slepi put stynkynge thynges unto hys nose to waken hym therewith."

There is much talk in the old herbals of "degrees," such

The vertues of Kebuli.

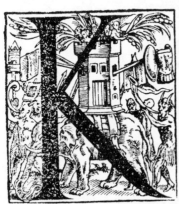

EBVLI purge fleme/increafe a mans reafon and vnderftandinge/ and helpe the memo ye/ and ftoppe the rewme/they fcoure the ftomach and ftrengthen/it quickeneth the eye fight and other fenfes/and are good for the dropfey and old agues. The pouder of the Indianes and the kebuli maye be taken from ij. ʒ to iiij. ʒ/ & the broth of the infufion of them maye be take from iiij.ʒ vnto xx. but he that taketh them/ muft not take them whiles the North winde bloweth / and muft eat no fifhe. The fodden broth of thefe do ftoppe more then the infufion/ whiche is onelye preffed out without fethinge.

FIGURE 68. Kebuli (text and decorative initial). Kebuli or Mirobalanes were commonly termed Indian almonds, and belong to the genus Terminalia, which has over 100 species. Those used in medieval medicine produced a dry, plumlike fruit with an edible kernel. The name Kebuli appears to refer to Kabul in Afghanistan as the point of origin. The plants were considered to be purgatives, especially of phlegm and melancholy. (From William Turner's *A New Herball*. Collen, A. Birckman, 1568. Original size 5 ⁵/₁₆″ wide × 2 ¹³/₁₆″ high.)

as dry and cold in the third degree, or warm and moist in the second. This goes back to the ancient Greek theory of four elements, four qualities, and four humours. Perhaps the clearest definition is Turner's, couched though it is in his unruly spelling:

A degre is as littell understanded as it is greatlye occupied in al mennis mouthes. A degre is in Latin *gradus*, and it commeth of *gradior*, to go, and is named in Greke *apostasis*, that is a standinge or going away from. The cause of the name is this: There are certeyne herbes that are temperate yt is of a mere qualitie or propertie betwene hote and cold, and are neither notablie hote nor cold. And if any herbe departe from the temperate herbes toward heat, and is sensible felt a littel hote, it is called hote in the first degre, and if it be a littel hoter, it is called hote in ye second degre, as though it had made two steppes or departinges from temperate, If an herbe be very hote, it may be called hote in the third degre. If it be so hote as it can be, then it is called hote in the fourth degre, and so ye maye understand the degrees of cold, moyst and drye herbes.

The terms hot, cold, etc. refer to effects rather than temperature or moisture content. The theory may have been founded on incomplete data, but nonetheless most herbs or substances that are assigned the fourth degree are either poisonous or violently harmful in their effects. Opium is cold and dry in the fourth degree, and poisonous mushrooms moist and cold in the same. Spurge, which is one of the poisonous *Euphorbias,* is hot in the fourth, as poison ivy would be if the old herbalists had classified it. So, even when Turner was somewhat in error, his words still carried a certain amount of wisdom.

BIBLIOGRAPHIC NOTES

1st edition: Part 1 of the *New Herball,* 1551 by Steven Mierdman at London.
2nd edition: Part 2, 1562 by Arnold Birckman at Collen (Cologne).
3rd edition: Part 3 with Parts 1 and 2 added, corrected, and enlarged, 1568 by Arnold Birckman at Collen (Cologne).

For further details see Trimen and Thistleton-Dyer's *Flora of Middlesex,* London, 1869.

❧ 20 ☙

The *Kreütterbuch* of Adam Lonitzer

 TRICTLY speaking, Lonitzer's *Kreütterbuch* cannot be called a new or independent work in any sense. It is simply a result of a combination, made originally in 1533, when Christian Egenolph issued revised versions of *Der Gart* and Brunschwig's *Destillierbuch* in one publication. The text at that time was edited by the Town Physician of Frankfurt am Main, Dr. Eucharius Rösslin. On Rösslin's death the herbal portion of the work was reedited by Theodore Dorsten and entitled the *Botanicon,* probably to make it seem to be a new production. Both of these publications were brought together, reedited, and combined with Lonitzer's own contributions in 1557 as the *Kreütterbuch,* which is thus a third- or fourth-hand reworking of late 15th-century material.

Many of the illustrations for the *Kreütterbuch* were not original either, having been pirated from the *Herbarum* of Brunfels and the *Historia Stirpium* of Fuchs, not to mention a number of other sources. Egenolph had once been sued successfully by Johann Schott of Strassburg, and forced to sur-

156

render all the woodcuts that he had plagiarized. It was an expensive lesson, but was also one that Egenolph blithely ignored. Throughout his entire career he continued the same practice, which the casual attitudes of his time permitted him to do with almost complete impunity. The sin of his plagiarism was partially redeemed by the fact that his block-cutters had a fluid, decorative style that made for extremely attractive books, and that his books were available to the public at relatively low prices. Many of the editions were expertly colored with transparent washes of watercolor rather than the opaque pigments that so often disfigured hand-colored herbals of the incunabula era. (For that reason uncolored copies are generally more attractive to buyers in the rare-book market.) Egenolph was also shrewd in his choice of illustrators, engaging Hans Beham to adapt many of the botanical designs, and Hans von Weiditz for pictures of animals and genre scenes. Succeeding generations have granted their approval of Egenolph's taste, if not his methods, for his books still sell at auctions while other books remain unsold.

By 1557, the year the Kreütterbuch was published, Adam Lonitzer had been Egenolph's son-in-law for some four years, having married into the family on the day he obtained his doctorate at Mainz in 1553. Lonitzer had thus become one of the heirs to the Egenolph publishing house, a highly valuable 16th-century property. And its value increased when edition after edition of Lonitzer's herbal tumbled from the presses, for it was a book that caught the popular fancy and held it. In fact, from its first appearance in 1533 as Rösslin's herbal it enjoyed good sales and repeated printings until 1783, a run of 250 years.

Through the course of numerous editions Lonitzer's text was repeatedly rearranged, and it is impossible to speak of any one version as the standard one. Although there was a liberal sprinkling of the fabulous and fictitious in the *Kreütterbuch*, it also contained the more useful portions of

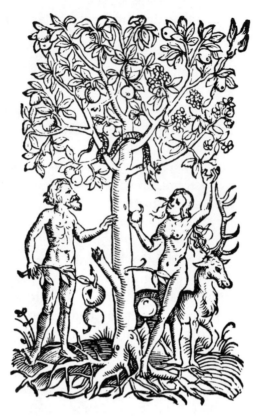

FIGURE 69. Adam and Eve and the Tree. Medicinal plants became a necessity to man once he became subject to illness and death as a result of the rash action of Adam and Eve. This picture of them in the act of losing their option on Paradise was a most appropriate opening for Lonitzer's section on remedial herbs. The stag is present as a symbol of lust, one of the other effects of man's loss of innocence. (From Lonitzer's *Kreuterbuch*. Frankfort, Egenolph, 1577. Original size 2 $\frac{1}{2}$" wide × 4 $\frac{5}{16}$" high.)

Brunschwig's writings on distillation, and so popularized a knowledge of distilling methods through all the German-speaking lands. Fuchs complained that it contained gross errors about the plants that were figured, but the voice of reason was drowned out by the applause of the crowd. If anything, its use of the fantastic added to its appeal, for

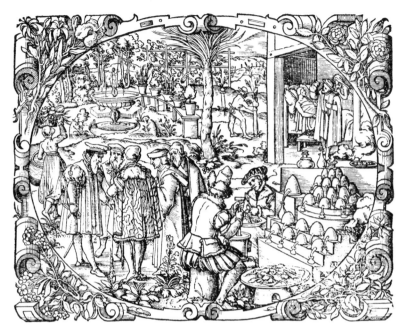

FIGURE 70. Medicine and herbs. The frontispiece to Lonitzer's *Kreuterbuch* clearly shows the importance of medicinal plants to the practice of medicine, or, as it was then termed, physic. The plants are seen about to be gathered from the garden, before which a group of physicians are shown in consultation. Immediately to the right of them an apothecary and his assistant are preparing and distilling herbs, while in the background a doctor administers them to his patient. (From Lonitzer's *Kreuterbuch*. Frankfort, Egenolph, 1577. Original size 5 ½″ wide × 4 ¼″ high.)

there were just enough exotic and magical ingredients to sustain the interest of the reader. For 20th-century readers this undoubtedly gives it a quaint and medieval charm, but for those who took its advice seriously some of the consequences must have been painful. On the other hand, some of the more outrageous remedies were perfectly safe, since their ingredients were often unprocurable.

The bulk of the prescriptions were founded on traditions that were not merely old but ancient. Claus Nissen points out a curious parallel between the use of *Ricinus*, the castor bean, in the Ebers Papyrus of c.1550 B.C., and in

Lonitzer's *Kreütterbuch* of some 3,000 years later. Both speak of its laxative properties, the use of its oil to cure itch, sores, and herpes when applied as a plaster, and the use of its pounded leaves to heal external ulcers. This is just one example among many of the persistence of herbal lore which passes almost unaltered from one generation to the next. The only point of difference in this case is that the ancient Egyptian work also recommends crushing the seeds, mixing them with grease, and anointing a woman's head to make her hair grow. It does not specify whether this would cure baldness, or simply act to encourage a more luxuriant and shinier growth.

Lonitzer's *Kreütterbuch* also perpetuated the myth of the

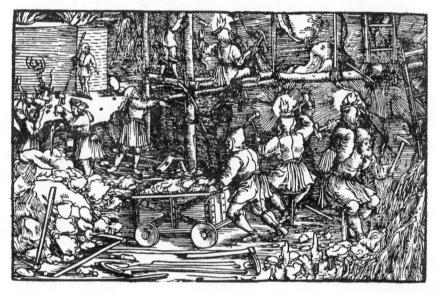

FIGURE 71. Mining scene. Lonitzer's book on stones and minerals as remedies was illustrated with this scene in a German mine. Within these burrows the first railways developed; handcarts were pushed about on metal rails. Mines were hazardous places to work, what with fumes from smelters (as in the upper left corner), rickety scaffolding and supports, and the ever-present danger of explosions and fires because of the presence of open flames on the miners' headgear. (From Lonitzer's *Kreuterbuch*. Frankfort, Egenolph, 1577. Original size 6 1/8" wide × 3 3/4" high.)

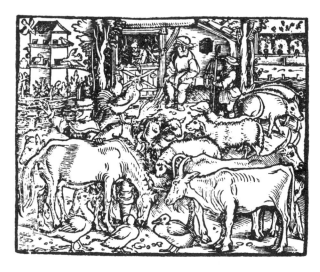

FIGURE 72. Barnyard. This cut heads Lonitzer's discussion of remedies derived from animals, and typifies the kind of medieval farmyard that was found among the more prosperous German farmers. Since the era was one of great inflation it is doubtful that this scene of peace and plenty was very common. The abundance of livestock and poultry reflects the fact that meat, not vegetables, formed the larger part of the diet. (From Lonitzer's *Kreuterbuch*. Frankfort, Egenolph, 1577. Original size 4 ¼″ wide × 3 ⁵/₁₆″ high.)

Barnacle Goose, reputedly born of rotting wood floating in the sea. The legend had supposedly been killed off with finality by Fabio Colonna in 1592, but it remained untouched in the Lonitzer text until the last edition of 1783. So did the tale of the Bezoar stone, that miraculous antidote to poison which was chiefly to be found within the stomach of a deer. Deer were supposed to be fond of killing snakes and then eating them. After so dining they went to a stream or pond and stayed there until the snake's venom was purged through their eyes. The presence of the stone in the deer's stomach or intestinal tract was supposedly the means by which the poison was driven off, and its life preserved. Such stones, or concretions, do exist. They are compounds of lime and magnesium phosphate that are found in several animals besides deer. They were usually placed in goblets to protect one from poisoned wine. Scrapings of the stone were also given in wine to cure internal ailments that supposedly had been caused by toxic substances. They were in vogue in Europe from the 12th century onwards, and there was quite a market for them in the time of Louis XIV, when medically useful stones sold for fifty times the price of an emerald of equal size. Poorer patients rented them by the day if they could not afford to buy them outright. There were both soluble and insoluble types. Elizabeth I of England owned a rather large one set in gold, which became part of the Crown jewels that passed to James I. Even as late as the 19th century the Bezoar was still in use, for the Shah of Persia presented Napoleon I with four of them, perhaps having heard of the Emperor's formidable roster of ailments, internal and otherwise.

With material of that sort it is small wonder that the *Kreütterbuch* endured so long. Its Arabian Nights aura may not have made for very many cures, but it did enliven many an evening with entertaining reading.

BIBLIOGRAPHIC NOTES

1st edition: 1557 by Christian Egenolffs Erben (Egenolph's Heirs) at Frankfort am Main. 708 woodcuts.

Subsequent editions from the same press in 1560–64 and 1569. In 1573 Martin Lechler issued an edition at Frankfort am Main which was followed by six more in 1577, 1578, 1582, 1587, 1593, and 1598. Three more by Sigismund Latomus of Frankfort am Main appeared in 1604–9 and 1616. Matthew Kempffer of Frankfort am Main produced two in 1630 and 1650. At Ulm two editions were printed by Matthew Wagner in 1674 and 1679. Another edition at Ulm by Daniel Bartholomä in 1713, and three more at Ulm by Daniel Bartholomä und Sohn in 1737, 1765, and 1770. Last edition by Joseph Wolffischen of Augsburg in 1783.

◄§ 21 ɮ►

The *Commentarii* of Pier Andrea Mattioli

N E of the most famous herbalists of the 16th century was Pier Andrea Mattioli, whose commentaries on Dioscorides made his name a household word throughout Europe. Born at Siena in 1501, he was educated at Venice and Padua. His father intended him to study law there, but Mattioli developed a distaste for it and determined to follow his father's profession, medicine. Unluckily, Mattioli's schooling was broken off because of the death of his father. But despite his early departure, the faculty awarded him his doctorate anyway, on the basis of his conduct and general merit.

The following two decades brought mixed blessings for Mattioli. He acquired an ample practice in Siena, but left there for Rome, where he remained for six or seven years until the barbarous sack of that city in 1527 by a rabble of mercenaries. Mattioli was fortunate enough to live through it and make his way to Valle Anania, near Trent, where he became very popular with the townspeople and stayed for fourteen years or more. He was next appointed Public Physician of Gorizia, from which he was called to Prague in 1555 to be the personal physician of the Archduke Maximilian. One wonders what he might have accomplished if he had had time to complete his medical studies at Padua.

Along the way Mattioli had developed a keen interest in the *Materia medica* and, like other physicians of his time, he sought to reconcile the teachings of Dioscorides with the innovations of the Arabs, the School of Salerno, and the botanical discoveries arriving every day from the Orient, the Americas, and Europe itself. The result was a book written in Italian and published at Venice in 1544 by Nicolo de Bascarini. Other editions followed, and in 1554 the prestigious Venetian press of Vincent Valgrisi brought out the first Latin edition of the work, illustrated with 562 woodcuts. It was an imposing production of an important work, and made Mattioli's name known throughout Europe. It aroused special interest in Prague, since one year after the book appeared Mattioli was invited there by the Holy Roman Emperor, Ferdinard I, to treat his son, the Archduke Maximilian. He continued his attachment to the Imperial Court in Vienna and Prague for over twenty years. Retiring to Trent in 1577, he died shortly afterwards, the victim of a plague. Mattioli was married twice and had several children, only one of whom followed the family calling by becoming physician to the Elector of Saxony.

Mattioli must have had an engaging personality up through his middle years, as is shown by the popular reaction when a fire destroyed all of his furnishings at Gorizia. The populace flocked as one to his aid the very next day. They presented him with goods and money, a year's salary was advanced to him, and he ended up richer than before the fire. But his obsession with his work on Dioscorides, a self-imposed task that consumed every spare moment, may well have warped his character later on. He set out to be the supreme authority of Dioscorides, and gradually reached a state where he would tolerate neither rivals nor corrections,

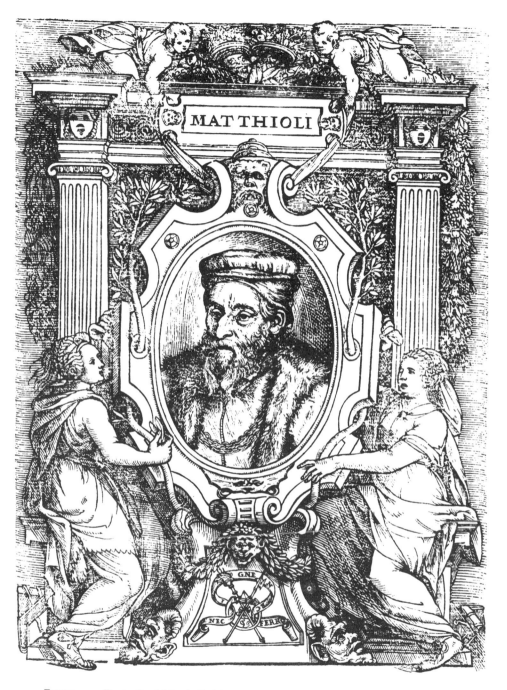

FIGURE 73. Portrait of Mattioli. Mattioli's portrait from the first Bohemian edition of his work, printed in 1562, shows him as physician to the Holy Roman Emperor, whose court was then located in the city of Prague. His motto, behind crossed torch and axe, reads *Nec igne, nec ferro* (Neither fire nor iron), referring to his preference for medication over surgical methods in order to effect his cures. (From Mattioli's *Herbarz: ginak Bylinář* . . . Prague, G. Melantrich, 1562. Original size 6 ⅛" wide × 8 ¼" high.)

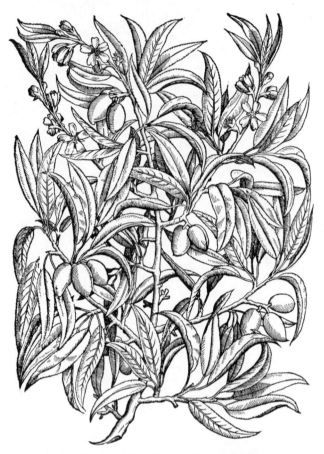

FIGURE 74. Almonds. From ancient times almonds were recommended as a cataplasm for removing spots from the skin, and if 5 or 7 were eaten before a drinking bout they were thought to prevent drunkenness. While growing, the almond looks much like an unripe apricot, and has a some-what leathery outer hull that splits in the fall to release the familiar pitted inner hull with its edible kernel. (From Mattioli's *Herbarz: ginak Bylinář* . . . Prague, G. Melantrich, 1562. Original size 6 1/8" wide × 8 5/8" high.)

even when they appeared in the most courteous guise. From his post at the Imperial Court he wielded immense influence throughout the European medical community, and some doctors soon discovered that his reach was long, indeed.

In 1565 a newly revised and augmented edition of his *Commentarii* was issued at Venice by the Valgrisi press. It

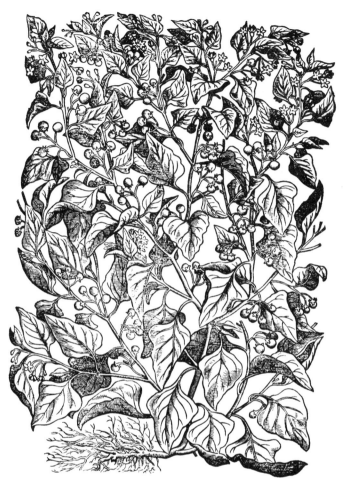

FIGURE 75. Garden Nightshade. The leaves of Garden Nightshade (*Solanum nigrum*) were used to cure headache, erysipelas, and shingles by external application. A poisonous principle present in the green parts of the plant, and to a lesser extent in the berries, varies in intensity at different seasons. It was called Garden Nightshade from its habit of springing up in or nearby cultivated places. (From Mattioli's *Herbarz: ginak Bylinář* . . . Prague, G. Melantrich, 1562. Original size 6″ wide × 8 ¹/₂″ high.)

bore some magnificent large woodcuts that carried that graphic technique to its utmost limits. In the preface, Mattioli praises the artists responsible, Giorgio Liberale and Wolfgang Meyerpeck, but then proceeds to inveigh against any physician or naturalist who dared disagree with him. Some of these, such as Amatus Lusitanos (Joam R. Amato), had been subjected to his abuse even earlier. Through charges levelled by Mattioli, Amatus (whose name Mattioli persisted in altering to Amathus, meaning simpleton) was hunted from place to place by the Inquisition. He finally obtained refuge in a Jewish colony in Salonica, but lost his livelihood, his reputation, and the manuscript of a translation of Avicenna that he had nearly completed.

Another victim of Mattioli's wrath was Luigi Anguillara (Luigi Squalermi), who was driven from his seat at the University of Padua. More fortunate than Amatus, he had friends at Ferrara and is rumored to have been given a professorship there, although Mattioli did succeed in clouding his name for a little over 200 years. The famous Conrad Gesner was also rebuked, as were Marant and Wieland, two other reputable medical men of the day. It was difficult to avoid conflict with Mattioli, for in his *Apologia adversus Amathum Lusitanum* and its sequel the *Censura* he compiled a list of 121 plants that he said he would battle over should anyone not accept his identifications.

Yet for all his bluster Mattioli did not have an expert knowledge of plants, nor were the working methods used for his *Commentarii* beyond reproach. He kept no specimens and, as a consequence, had no means of checking the accuracy of illustrations or of plant identifications offered to him. Botanists have noted that in some cases false pictures were given to him, and succeeded in being used because he was ignorant of the facts. There was reason enough for this, since many hitherto unknown plants were being introduced from just about everywhere. Some that were submitted to Mattioli, especially those from places such as Turkey, were dried and had to be reconstituted by soaking before the artists could draw them. Under such circumstances error was bound to occur.

Over the years, he continued to rework his text and

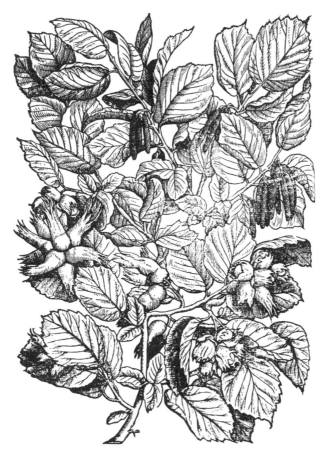

FIGURE 76. Hazelnuts. Hazelnuts were recommended by Dioscorides for restoring fallen hair, for deepening gray eyes to a black color (only feasible with children), and for curing an old cough. Some herbalists regarded them as useful in stopping dysentery, while others considered them to be a cause of it. (From Mattioli's *Herbarz: ginak Bylinář* . . . Prague, G. Melantrich, 1562. Slightly reduced from original size, 6 ⅛" wide × 8 ⅝" high.)

ended by completely overwhelming the contributions of Dioscorides with his annotations and commentary. As an example, Dioscorides' preface occupies 1 folio page, whereas Mattioli's runs to 14. Elsewhere, and these are purely random examples, Dioscorides' 12 lines on galingale, an aro-

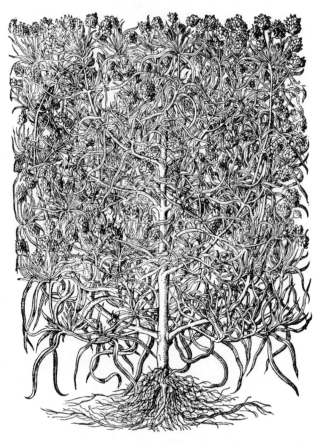

FIGURE 77. Psyllium. This depiction of Psyllium (*Plantago psyllium*) is one of the most dazzling bits of virtuosity in Mattioli's herbal. Difficult to draw, the complexities of cutting the design into wood are even greater, as can be seen in this majestic tangle. Psyllium was known as Fleawort because the seeds looked like fleas. In Latin it was called Pulicaria. Used in modern times as a mild laxative, it was formerly prescribed for relieving fevers and burning sensations of the inner parts. (From Mattioli's *Herbarz: ginak Bylinář* . . . Prague, G. Melantrich, 1562. Original size 6 1/4" wide × 8 5/8" high.)

matic sedge (*Cyperus rotundus*), are supplemented with 55 by Mattioli. On plantain, Dioscorides has 4 page-width lines, folio size (about equal to 8 or 10 of an octavo page), while Mattioli occupies another 30. In one of the most extensive expansions, on acorus (*Iris pseudacorus*), Mattioli adds

140 lines to the original 7 of Dioscorides. The commentary obviously outweighed its subject, and became a record of all the plants known to Mattioli. Not much, of course, is useful to modern botany, save for original descriptions of plants that were then new in Europe.

One other blemish on Mattioli's career is his experimentation on condemned criminals to determine if Monkshood (*Aconitum napellus*) was more poisonous than other aconites. It is said that some of the experiments ended with fatalities. Nothing, not even Auschwitz, is new under the sun.

All in this compendious and sumptuous herbal reflects the violence and the beauty of its age. It held great appeal for its readers, and was translated from the original Italian into Latin, French, German, and Czech. Altogether about 45 editions were printed. We have the word of the printer Valgrisi that the early editions obtained a sale of 32,000 copies, and he himself printed fourteen editions in all.

Mattioli's portrait in one of the Latin editions bears two mottoes, one in Greek, "Dyskola ta Kala" (ΔΥΣΚΟΛΑ ΤΑ ΚΑΛΑ), and the other in Latin, "Nec igne nec ferro." The first translates "The good things are difficult," referring to the art of healing. The second, "Neither fire nor iron," refers to his preference for physic, in which those two tools of the surgeon are shunned like the plague. Noble sentiments, but the portrait that accompanies them shows a face that seems touched with both iron and fire. There was probably more than one sigh of relief when in 1577 the word came from Trent that the great Mattioli had been felled by the plague.

BIBLIOGRAPHIC NOTES

1st edition: 1544 by Nicolo de Bascarini at Venice. In Italian, no illustrations. Other editions without illustration in 1547, 1548,

1549, 1552, by various Italian printers. Three illustrated editions, small woodcuts, by Valgrisi of Venice in 1555, 1563, 1568. Three others by Valgrisi with large cuts in 1570, 1581, 1604.

1st Latin edition: 1554 by Vincent Valgrisi at Venice. Four others by Valgrisi in 1558, 1559, 1570, 1596, all with small cuts.

Latin Editions by Valgrisi with large cuts in 1565, 1569, 1583. The Latin *Commentarii* also appear in the *Opera omnia* of 1598 and 1674. Last Latin edition in 1744 by Nicolaum Pezzanam at Venice.

1st French edition: 1561 by Gabriel Cotier at Lyon. Small woodcuts. Other French editions, all with small cuts, from various printers in 1572, 1605, 1642, 1655, 1680.

1st German edition: 1562 by Georgen Melantrich at Prague. Under title: *New Kräuterbuch*. Large woodcuts.

Other German editions, all with small cuts, done at Frankfort am Main in 1590, 1598, 1600, 1611, 1626. Last German edition 1678 at Basel.

1st Czech (Bohemian) edition: 1562 by Girkiia Melantryka (Georg Melantrich) at Prague. This was the first use of the large woodcuts. Two further Czech editions in 1566 and 1596 with small woodcuts.

~§ 22 §~

The *Crüÿdeboeck* of Rembert Dodoens

H E Spanish Netherlands in the 16th century was hardly the time nor the place to provide the calm and uninterrupted quiet so necessary for the advancement of learning. Yet a number of scholars, including the famed anatomist, Vesalius, and the botanists Clusius, L'Obel, and Dodoens, developed there. These last three continued the tradition established by Bock. They investigated the local flora and shattered the traditional notion that the plants of Europe made but one indivisible flora, all perfectly known and described by the ancients. L'Obel investigated the plants of southern France, especially about Narbonne, Clusius studied those of Austria-Hungary, and Dodoens studied those of the Netherlands. Their work formed the basis for the later systems of Cesalpino, Bauhin, and Linnaeus, which culminated in the formation of modern botanical taxonomy.

Dodoens was born in Flanders in 1517 in the town of Mechlin, now Malines, of a well-to-do family whose members included physicians and magistrates. He studied

173

medicine at Louvain, where he graduated in 1535 at the age of eighteen. Apparently feeling too young to enter immediately into practice, he travelled through Italy, France, and Germany. In all probability he used the trip to further his medical studies, though he makes no mention in his memoirs of what he did during that time. Not until 1548 is there a clear record of Dodoens' activities, for in that year he wrote a book, *De sphaera*, on cosmography and astronomy, and was appointed Town Physician of Malines. He remained a citizen of that town until 1574, when he departed for Vienna and Prague.

Dodoens' cousin, the Councilor Hopper, Administrator of Affairs in the Netherlands, had proposed in 1568 that he become physician to Philip II, but Dodoens preferred to remain at home. He had by that time settled down with his wife, Catherine S'Bruynen, and five children, and was the author of several botanical works already published. In 1572, however, the idyllic picture changed. His wife died, and a few months later the town of Malines was put to the torch and sword by the Spaniards. Dodoens' house was pillaged, and all he had was destroyed. Hopper once again renewed the offer that he become physician to Philip II, but Dodoens wanted a good deal of distance between himself and anything Spanish. His friend Clusius then obtained for him the post of personal physician to the Holy Roman Emperor, Maximilian II, which had been vacated by Mattioli on his retirement. Dodoens accepted, and from 1574 through 1578 filled that office in Vienna and Prague. Maximilian had died in the meantime, and had been succeeded by Rudolph II, who continued Dodoens' appointment. The atmosphere in the Royal Court at Prague was not to Dodoens' liking, so he resigned and went to live in Cologne, where he published several botanical and medical writings. Later he spent a brief sojourn in Malines to straighten out matters pertaining to his properties and estate. In 1582 the University of Ley-

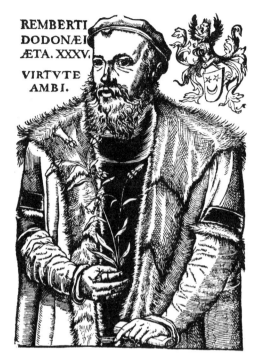

FIGURE 78. Portrait of Dodoens. At age 35, Dodoens was a man of virtue, as he was throughout all his life. The coat of arms with the two stars and crescent moon was that of his family. Dodoens is shown here two years before the appearance of his *Crüÿdeboeck* at Antwerp in 1554, a work now so excessively rare that only about 5 copies are known. (From *A Nievve Herball*. London, G. Dewes, 1578. Original size 3 ³/₈″ wide × 4 ⁷/₈″ high.)

den named him to their chair of botany, and he stayed there in that capacity until his death in 1585 at the age of 68.

The botanical work of Clusius, L'Obel, and Dodoens, although in separate volumes under their individual names, is so interrelated that it is difficult to know what to attribute to whom. They corresponded regularly, and shared their in-

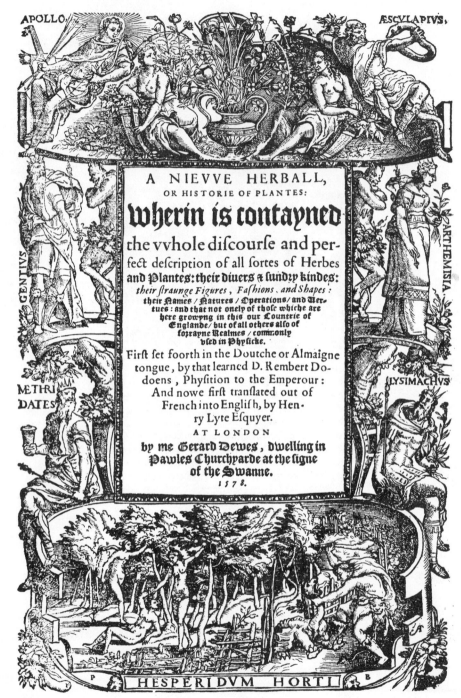

FIGURE 79.

formation, their publisher, and even the illustrations to their books. In point of fact the *Plantarum seu Stirpium icones* of Matthias L'Obel, published at Antwerp in 1581 by the Plantin press, is a compendium of all the illustrations that had appeared in the published botanical writings of all three authors. It is a massive, two-volume edition containing the entire repertoire of botanical woodcuts, some 2,173 of them, that belonged to the Plantin establishment. L'Obel's part in it was to arrange the cuts, provide them with Latin names, and compose an index wherein the Latin terms were given their Dutch, German, French, Italian, Spanish, Portuguese, and English equivalents. L'Obel's arrangement was an attempt, based on differences in leaf structures, to create a system of classification "according to their kind and their mutual relationship."

Dodoens' first botanical work of importance was the *Crüÿdeboeck*, published at Antwerp in 1554 by Jan vander Loë. This provided the basis for all of his further writings since his later works merely incorporated additions and changes that he made to the original during the rest of his lifetime. His work finally bore the title *Stirpium historiae in pemptades sex*, and was issued by Christophe Plantin of Antwerp in 1583, just two years before Dodoens' death. It is a heavy folio volume of nearly 900 pages, with some 1,309 woodcuts, six of them copies made from the illustrations to the *Juliana Anicia Codex* of Dioscorides.

The *Crüÿdeboeck* of 1554 borrowed heavily from the woodcuts made at Basle in 1545 to illustrate the octavo editions of Fuchs. Of the 707 cuts that appeared in vander Loë's

FIGURE 79. Title page of *A Nievve Herball*. Some 24 years after it first appeared, Dodoens' *Crüÿdeboeck* was translated into English by Henry Lyte, who avoided the pitfalls of the original Flemish by using a French version. The title page of the 1578 *Nievve Herball*, as Lyte called it, is seen here with its elaborate border presenting a veritable medical pantheon. (From Dodoens' *A Nievve Herball*. London, G. Dewes, 1578. Original size 6 1/8" wide × 10 3/16" high.)

edition, only about 170 were original. Such extensive borrowing, in fact, seems to have been the case for most of the published herbals of Dodoens.

The botanical historian, Ernst Meyer, credits Dodoens with advancing botany toward systematic classification, but Dodoens himself said that Dioscorides' plan was still the most practical. It classified plants according to their properties, and only secondarily according to form. Following that principle he condemned the Doctrine of Signatures, which stated that the form of a plant signified what it was to be used for.

Dodoens' scientific descriptions carried a certain touch of color and poetry that did not always facilitate his desire for clear and unequivocal statements. Concerning a vital element of plant morphology, he had this to say: "The flower we call the joy of trees and plants. It is the hope of fruits to come, for every growing thing, according to its nature, produces offspring and fruit after the flower. But flowers have their own special parts." Thus, standing on the brink of discovering the sexuality of plants, he failed to take the next step that would have brought him even greater fame.

Dodoens' *Crüÿdeboeck,* before it eventually metamorphosed into the *Pemptades,* grew in a rather piecemeal fashion. Perhaps best known to English readers is the translation made in 1578 by Henry Lyte. That in turn was made from the French translation by Clusius of the original Flemish *Crüÿdeboeck.* It is obvious that a Dodoens bibliography entails using several names for a central work that appeared in parts from time to time. The Lyte translation, known as *Nievve Herball, or Historie of Plantes* may well have supplied Shakespeare with much of the plant lore used in his plays. And the illustrations, used in all the successive publications, provided ample but low-paying work for the artists and engravers of the Plantin press. Dodoens' fellow townsman, Pieter van der Borcht, made the drawings for 12 to 13 sous each, and the engravers, Arnaud Nicolai and Gerard Jansen van Kampen, received about 7 sous for every block they cut.

It is a bit difficult to find a coherent system underlying Dodoens' arrangement of plants, since its plan combines the dissimilar ones of Theophrastus and Dioscorides. Book I of the eventual *Pemptades* lists herbaceous plants in alphabetical order. Book II is on flowers used in garlands and bouquets, or for their aroma, and also treats of the umbellifers. Book III is on roots, vines, poisonous plants, and cryptogams. Book IV concerns cereals, leguminous plants, and those of the marsh and seashore. Book V treats of edible plants, and Book VI is about shrubs, trees, forest trees, and evergreens. Throughout the work, broad classifications *do* become visible, and some genuine natural relationships are established. Using hindsight it is simple enough to see the shortcomings of Dodoens' herbal, but considering the confusion that reigned in the botanical knowledge of his age, it must be admitted that he made positive contributions. Certainly he deserves the tribute on his tomb in the Church of St. Peter in Leyden. There, beneath his coat of arms, two golden stars, and a crescent moon on a field of blue, is carved the following inscription:

> To An Excellent Man, of the Greatest Worth, Rembert Dodoens, Doctor to the Emperors Maximilian II and Rudolph II, Physician and Councilor, Whose Learning and Writing in Things Astronomical, Botanical and Medical Brought Him Fame, A Onetime Senior of the Leyden Academy, This Memorial from the people of Holland to the Professor of Medicine Who Died Happily on the 10th Day of March, 1585, at His Age of 68, Rembert Dodoens.

Too bad there was no repetition of the gesture Dodoens made at the funeral of his wife. To insure that the town of Malines would hold her in kind memory, he honored her by making a public distribution of strawberries and wine in her name. The same would have been botanically apt as a memorial to him.

BIBLIOGRAPHIC NOTES

1st edition: 1554 by Jan vander Loë at Antwerp. 715 woodcuts. A second edition in 1563 from the same press had 841 woodcuts.

1st English edition: 1578 by Gerard Dewes at London (but printed at Antwerp by Henry Loë). Translated by Henry Lyte. 870 woodcuts. Other editions in 1586, 1595, 1600. Unillustrated edition in 1619 titled *A Nievve Herball.*

1st French edition: 1557 by Jean Loë at Antwerp. 840 woodcuts. Titled *Histoire des plantes.*

1st Latin edition: 1583 by Christophe Plantin at Antwerp. 1,309 woodcuts. Titled *Stirpium historiae Pemptades sex.* A second edition in 1616 by Balthasar and Johannes Moretus with 1,341 woodcuts.

◆§ 23 §◆

Thurneisser's *Historia*

HATEVER erroneous data marred the pages of most herbals was not a result of deliberate design, but rather a reflection of the learning and custom of an age. Leonhard Thurneisser's *Historia sive descriptio plantarum omnium,* however, is quite another matter, for there the intent was to impress, to deceive, and to sell. Gifted with a quick, perceptive mind, he learned quite soon in life that there were many gulls waiting, in fact longing, to be duped, and so he settled on his road to fortune.

Born at Basel in 1530, he became a skilful goldsmith (his father's trade), helped a local physician to gather herbs, and read to him from the writings of Paracelsus. No doubt it was then that he formed many of the astrological and alchemical notions that he later put into practice. At the age of 17, involved in debt through the actions of an unfaithful wife, he faked the alchemical production of gold by gilding a block of lead. It proved to be one of those bright ideas that should be avoided at any cost, for the substitution was discovered and Thurneisser had to escape across the border into Germany.

He took up his trade as a goldsmith at Strassburg and

later at Constance, manufactured mathematical instruments, and involved himself in metallurgy with such success that he was made director of the smelting works at Eberswold in the Tyrol. By then, 1558, he had married for the second time. His wife was a goldsmith's daughter who managed his affairs with skill and prudence.

For years afterwards his was a story of peace, prosperity, and plenty. He came under the patronage of the Archduke Ferdinand, and through his knowledge of metallurgy was made an examiner of mines in Bohemia and Hungary. Owing to his extravagant tastes, a lifelong habit, Thurneisser fell from royal favor and moved into other spheres of activity. A well-timed cure of the Margrave of Brandenburg launched him on a medical career, which he made as remunerative as possible. Thurneisser capitalized on the prevailing interest in astrology and alchemy, and was not averse to selling magical potions, amulets, and expensive gemstones as medicines to his wealthy clientele. His publications, and especially his manuscripts, fetched outrageous prices. In addition, he corresponded with the emperor Maximilian II and Queen Elizabeth I.

Eventually it ended as it had to end. His wife died, depriving him of her steadying influence, his cures came into question, his printing press and staff became a cumbersome expense, and Thurneisser found it necessary to leave his luxurious lifestyle in Berlin, where he had been long established. Returning to Basel, he married for the third time, but soon fled to Italy to get away from domestic troubles. He evidently attempted alchemy in Italy, where he reportedly converted half of an iron nail into gold. Nonetheless poverty overtook him, and he died penniless in a monastery in Cologne, after making the modest request that he be interred near Albert the Great.

Thurneisser's *Historia* was intended to treat of all known plants in a ten-volume set. However, only the first volume was published, and its botanical value, as well as its medical

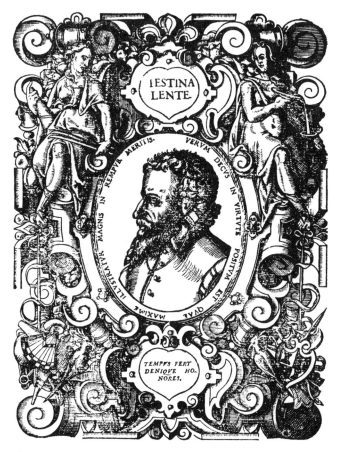

FIGURE 80. Portrait of Thurneisser. Like most scoundrels who seek to cozen their victims instead of forcibly plundering them, Thurneisser devised a camouflage of respectability for himself. Who could doubt the merits of a man whose portrait is so impressively presented? Thurneisser was a 16th-century master of the 20th-century art of public relations and image-making. (From Thurneisser's *Historia*. Berlin, M. Hentzske, 1578. Original size 5 $^7/_8''$ wide × 7 $^7/_8''$ high.)

value, was absolutely nil. An elaborate typographical production, with printed annotations in the margins, blocks of text inserted within other textual matter, lavish use of Hebrew and Greek characters, plus a host of astrological sym-

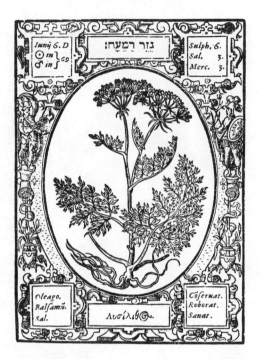

FIGURE 81. Umbellifer. Obviously this plant, because of its ribbed flower head, is of the order of
umbellifers. Some other members of the family are
parsley, carrots, Queen Anne's lace, and angelica.
Which particular umbellifer the picture intends to
show, however, is left uncertain. Nor do the labels
in Hebrew and Greek, with accompanying Latin
and astrological tags, help the reader very much, for
they were put there to mystify rather than inform.
(From Thurneisser's *Historia*. Berlin, M. Hentzske,
1578. Original size 3 ⁵/₁₆" wide × 4 ⁹/₁₆" high.)

bols, diagrams, and plant illustrations, the *Historia* delights
the eye while offering little but offense to the mind. The
descriptions of distillation methods are illustrated with
horses, giraffes, fish, bulls, and other animals which often
merge with the distilling apparatus itself. Only um-
belliferous plants are depicted, but it is next to impossible to
identify their species through the pictures.

The entire emphasis is on the astrological governance of

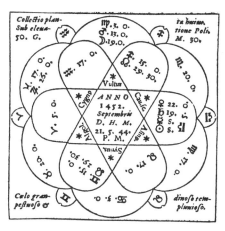

FIGURE 82. An astrological chart. Scattered
throughout Thurneisser's *Historia* are numerous horoscopes with their arcane symbols. The divisions on the left side of the
diagram, marked with the V-like sign of
Aries, represent the ascendant house of the
zodiac, and the twelve houses were arranged
in counterclockwise order from it. Its major
purpose was to baffle the uninitiated. (From
Thurneisser's *Historia.* Berlin, M. Hentzske,
1578. Original size 3 $\frac{1}{4}$" wide × 3 $\frac{1}{4}$" high.)

the plants, and the proper time to pick them and prepare
them for particular diseases and uses. Plants are classified as
male, female, and children, depending upon the degree of
strength and activity they manifest. Herbs used to cure
males are to be gathered when the sun or moon is in Sagit-
tarius, Aquarius, or at least in Leo. Those intended to cure
women are to be plucked preferably in Virgo, otherwise
Taurus or Cancer. All is murkiness, with lots of lofty phrases
intended to mystify. The formula worked as successfully
then as it unfortunately does now.

    Thurneisser was by no means unique. He had a coun-
terpart in Bartholomaeus Carrichter, who published another
astrological herbal in 1575 at Strassburg. Carrichter had also
been able to impress royalty, for he was physician to the
Holy Roman Emperors Maximilian II and Ferdinand I. It is a

cliché that the state they ruled was neither holy, Roman, nor an empire despite its name. It seems equally trite that those who ruled it had to suffer, literally, from a lack of medical attention at the hands of such quacks as Carrichter and Thurneisser.

The astrological school of medical botany carried on down into the 17th century, when one of its most famous exponents, Nicholas Culpeper (1616–54), did Londoners a great favor in 1649 by translating the *London Physical Directory*, long used by the physicians of that city. When, thanks to the translation, the populace realized how antique their prescriptions were, and how seldom of real use, reforms were undertaken and an official pharmacopeia was brought into being.

Astrological herbalism, however, did not die out after Culpeper. It is with us still, and will probably continue, blithely disregarding the dictates of common sense. It forms a colorful if somewhat raffish chapter in herbal and botanical history. About all that can be said for it is that its prescriptions in the past, when gemstones were powdered to be given in potions, helped to recycle and circulate wealth. And sometimes, as in the sequence of events set off when Culpeper revealed the medieval medical arsenal of 17th-century London doctors, a long-needed reform was brought about. Folly does occasionally commit such excessive absurdity that common sense is forced, for the moment, to rescue mankind from itself.

BIBLIOGRAPHIC NOTES

1st edition: 1578 by Michael Hentzske at Berlin.
2nd edition: 1578 by same printer at same place, but translated from Latin into German; titled *Historia und Beschreibung Influentischer, Elementischer und Natürlicher Wirckungen aller fremdem und heimischen Erdegewechsen. . . .*
Last edition: 1587 for Joannem Gymnicum at Cologne.

৵ 24 ৵

The *Herbario Nuovo* of Castore Durante

EITHER botanical science nor its illustration owe much to the *Herbario Nuovo*, yet it possesses an undeniable charm that brought it great popularity in Italy. The author, Castore Durante, was physician to Pope Sixtus the Fifth and had studied at the Sapienza in Rome. He was born about 1523 at Gualdo near Spoleto, some fifty miles northeast of Rome in the province of Umbria. He died at Viterbo in 1590, at the age of about 67. It is known that he was a physician, had a reputation as a poet, and was something of a botanist, but other particulars of his life remain obscure.

The *Herbario* was first published in Rome in 1585, only five years before his death, and thus would seem to be the result of his life's work. It presents all of the medicinal plants of Europe and the East and West Indies that were then known. The arrangement is the familiar alphabetical one, which at the time was about to be discarded because it separated related items. The illustrations, largely adapted from Fuchs and Mattioli, often incorporate bits of landscape

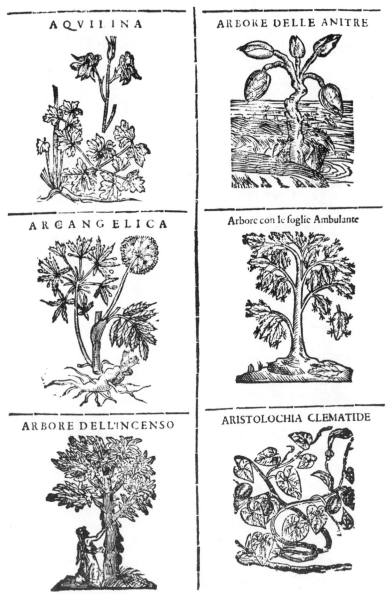

FIGURE 83. Six plants from the *Herbario Nuovo*. An appendix to Durante's book sought to save space by grouping blocks of the illustrations on one page. Aquilina or Columbine made a lotion for sore throats; the Arbore delle Anitre was the legendary Barnacle Goose Tree; Arcangelica was used in many remedies, syrups, and confections; Arbore con la figlia Ambulante was thought to have leaves that walked; Arbore dell' Incenso was the Incense Tree; and Aristolochia Clematide was the familiar Birthwort. (From Durante's *Herbario Nuovo*. Rome, Bonfadino and Diani, 1585. Original size 6 $^1/_2$" wide × 10" high.)

C A M P H O R A.

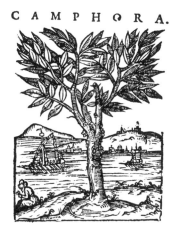

FIGURE 84. Camphora. For centuries Europeans had been in doubt about the origin of camphor. Durante shows it here, correctly, as a gummy exudation from a tree, a fact that came to light because of the many explorations of the 15th and 16th centuries. One of the Lauraceae, it is related to cinnamon and avocados, and was used externally to relieve the heat of fever and inflammation. Moth preventative cabinets made of its wood resisted the inroads of worms and borers. (From Durante's *Herbario Nuovo*. Rome, Bonfadino and Diani, 1585. Original size 2″ wide × 2 ⅞″ high.)

with men or animals pursuing various activities in the background. Either Durante was somewhat conservative in his outlook on *materia medica,* or else he enjoyed imitating the medieval style of Macer Floridus, for many of the simples that he mentions are headed by a Latin verse such as Macer used when describing the medicinal values of a plant. Following the verse he gives plant names in Greek, Latin, and Italian, adding German, Arabic, Spanish, or dialect names when they were known to him. Synonyms from foreign languages were by now a popular feature in herbals, following a fashion that had begun with Dioscorides and which was greatly amplified by Fuchs, Turner, Dodoens, and others.

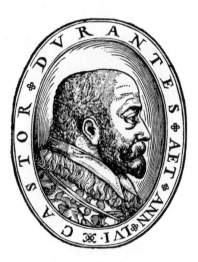

FIGURE 85. Portrait of Durante. Castor Durante, author of the *Herbario Nuovo,* probably the most popular herbal written in Italian is seen here at the age of 56. Although this is not a full-length representation of him, he seems to have been a rather thickset man. Befitting his position as doctor to the Pope, he is dressed in a robe of rich brocade. (From Durante' *Herbario Nuovo.* Venice, Li Sessa, 1602. Original size 3″ wide × 3 7/8″ high.)

Durante then went on to name each species, its time of flowering or ripening, and its medicinal qualities and uses. The work differed little in substance from earlier productions such as *Der Gart* or the *Hortus sanitatis,* and was a handy summation of the 16th-century herbal repertoire. The complete but concise discussions probably account for much of the great popularity that the work enjoyed. It was even printed in Germany in 1609 at Frankfort am Main as the *Hortulus sanitatis . . . Ein . . . Gahrtlin der Gesundheit,* an archaic title that fitted its somewhat outmoded material. No credit was given to Durante as author, but he was long since past caring, having died almost twenty years before. The situation was ideal for a plagiarist.

OLIVA SALVATICA.

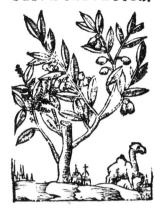

FIGURE 86. Wild olive. The olive tree was familiar throughout much of Italy, but here the presence of a camel hints that it had a Near Eastern origin. Durante remarks on the astringent quality of the leaves, which is quite different from the soothing, emollient effect of the oil from its fruits. The oil was used in treating skin diseases, and, when administered internally, was a good laxative as well as an antidote to irritant poisons. (From Durante's *Herbario Nuovo*. Rome, Bonfadino and Diani, 1585. Original size 2″ wide × 2 ⁷/8″ high.)

The *Herbario* has nearly a thousand chapters, each carrying a small woodcut just above the text. They were the work of Isabella Parasole, who made the designs, and Leonardo Norsino, who cut the blocks. While the basic character of the illustrations obviously derives from Fuchs and Mattioli, there are many original touches as well. For instance Squill, sometimes called the sea onion, is represented by a magnificent specimen riding the waves. It dwarfs a galleon that is weathering the seas in the background. The cut for Cinnamon shows a jovial, smiling sun shining brightly down on what may well be the Golden Horn. The view shows a range of hills and vaguely Oriental houses beyond a wide stretch of water containing oared galleys and galleons under sail. Directly in the foreground, resting to one side of the cinnamon tree, is a Turk wearing a turban and gazing out over the water. Elsewhere we see the Arbutus or Strawberry tree, beneath which a seated shepherd is piping happily on a flute. On a somewhat more sinister note, there is *Fongo corraloide,* probably *Amanita muscaria,* a bright red poisonous mushroom. It is represented by a little drama played out before a nearby palace or monastery, wherein a man and a snake are flying from each other with the greatest of haste. From the violent thrashing of the snake, though it appears uninjured, it seems to have had the worst of the situation.

There are a number of other such touches, most of them of a gently humanizing nature, or with a poetic touch of fancy such as a weeping tree. It is likely that these delightful little illustrations are what kept Durante's *Herbario* alive for over 130 years, despite its outmoded format.

BIBLIOGRAPHIC NOTES

1st edition: 1585 by Bartholomeo Bonfadino and Tito Diani at Rome. A second printing in the same year was done by Bonfadino and Diani for Jacomo Bericchia and Jacomo Tornierij. Other editions followed in 1602, 1612, 1617, 1636, 1666, 1667, 1684, 1717, and 1718. The last edition, in 1718, was printed at Venice by Michele Hertz.

A German translation was printed in 1609 at Frankfort am Main by Nicolaum Hoffmann. Edited by Petrum Uffenbachium.

~§ 25 ᖒ

The *Phytognomonica* of Giambattista Porta

CIENCE and magic competed to dominate the minds of men through the 16th century. For every advance, as in the case of Bock or Turner, there was a balancing regression, such as the fraudulence of Thurneisser. Sometimes, however, both features were combined in a single man, as was the case with Giambattista Porta, the Neapolitan wonder-worker.

Born at Naples about 1535, Porta took an early interest in the study of nature, was well educated, and wrote essays in both Italian and Latin by the age of ten. Later, under the auspices of his uncle, he travelled through Spain, France, and Italy, visiting famous libraries and learned men in his relentless search for knowledge. He had a genuine passion for finding out the why of things, for ferreting out the secrets of nature, and sometimes that deep and sincere desire trapped him into being overly credulous. Because he had received the tale on seemingly reliable authority, Porta believed that poisoned elephants sought out the plant called aloes, and thereby purged the venom from their bodies. The only difficulty was that aloes then came principally from the Island of Socotra, which was destitute of elephants.

At Naples, Porta, together with his brother Gian Vincenzo, gathered materials for a small museum (probably a cabinet of curiosities somewhat smaller than the famous collection of Ferrante Imperato) and offered its use to other scientists. He also established an organization, the Otiosi (Men of Leisure), which held meetings at his home and became the forerunner of such scientific groups as the Accademia dei Lincei and England's Royal Society. The Otiosi later called themselves the Accademia Secretorum Naturae, and made membership contingent upon the contribution of some new fact or discovery useful to science, medicine, or philosophy. Porta also attempted to create an interest in private schools for science, and tried to promote the concept of public academies.

Quite naturally all this activity brought him to the attention of the ecclesiastical authorities, and Porta and his circle were reported unfavorably to Pope Paul V. The court of Rome ordered him to disband his society, even though he demonstrated that its purpose was opposed to witchcraft. After all, there was no need to delve into nature, since revelation had provided man with the facts of his fall and redemption. Porta was obedient to the prohibition, but continued to permit his home to be a forum for the learned minds of his day. He became a member of the Accademia dei Lincei, which included Galileo and also Fabio Colonna, who was prominent in botanical circles. The Lincei derived their name and emblem from the lynx, an animal known for its clear and far-sighted vision, as well as its razor sharp claws that cut through to the most secret and well-guarded places to obtain nourishment.

Porta was truly more at home in the exact sciences of mathematics and physics than in the biological sciences. His *Elementa Curvilinea* and *De Refractione Optices* were both of

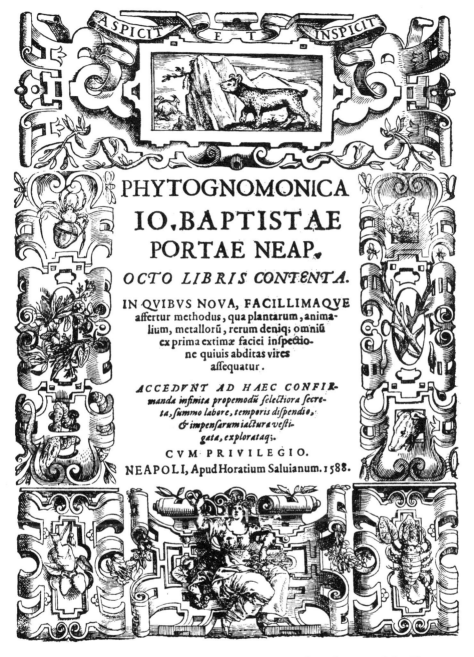

FIGURE 87. Title page of Porta's *Phytognomonica*. The title page of the *Phytognomonica* was a rather elaborate one, reflecting the importance of its author, who had already published many works of scientific value. The panel at top center shows a lynx, emblem of the Accademia Lincei, of which Porta was a member. Galileo and Colonna were fellow associates in that society. The words Aspicit-Inspicit mean "He looks at and looks within." (From Porta's *Phytognomonica*. Naples, H. Salviani, 1588. Original size 6 ³/₄" wide × 9 ⁹/₁₆" high.)

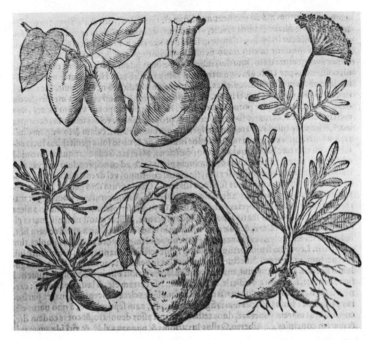

FIGURE 88. Heart plants. The Doctrine of Signatures is presented in the foreword to Book III of the *Phytognomonica*. There Porta states that the forms of plants reveal the purposes for which they are to be used. Hence peaches, citrons, and certain bulbous roots proclaim themselves as remedies for heart troubles and diseases because of their resemblance to a heart. (From Porta's *Phytognomonica*. Naples, H. Salviani, 1588. 6″ wide × 5 ¼″ high.)

genuine value, but his *De Humana Physiognomia* and the *Phytognomonica* seem to be the work of a fantasist, explaining character and purpose by means of external appearances. He also had a belief in natural astrology founded not on superstition but on the astronomical theories of Aristotle, wherein nature received its motivating force from the movement of the heavenly bodies. In Porta's own words on the subject,

> . . . whosoever is rightly seen in all these things [i.e., the effects of the stars and planets], he will ascribe all these inferiors [things happening below on earth] to the stars as

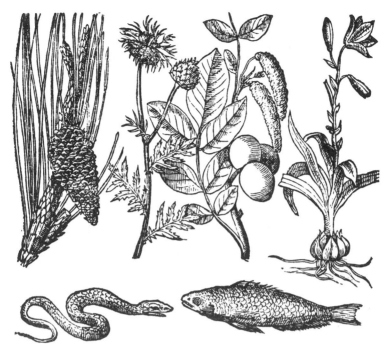

FIGURE 89. Plants for scaly diseases. According to the Doctrine of Signatures, scaly things such as pine-cones, thistles, catkins, and the overlapping skin on lily bulbs could be used to cure scaly conditions of the skin, especially any that were accompanied by slimy issues or sloughing. The snake and fish were added to show scaly skin. (From Porta's *Phytognomonica*. Naples, H. Salviani, 1588. Original size 6 ¼" wide × 5 ½" high.)

their causes; whereas if a man be ignorant hereof, he loseth the greatest part of the knowledge of secret operations and works of nature.

Imbued with such a viewpoint, and given his ample credulity, it is no surprise that he developed a theory like the Doctrine of Signatures. Quite simply this meant that the Creator had marked out a path for mankind in the treatment of disease and injury by placing a sign or hint on those natural products, mostly plants, which would be useful in healing them. Pine cones, lily bulbs, the flower heads of sca-

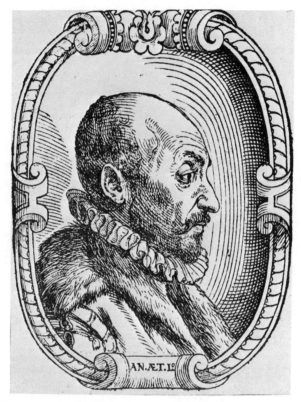

FIGURE 90. Portrait of Porta. This portrait of Giambattista Porta at age 50 appeared in his *Phytognomonica*, published at Naples in 1588. The work is famed for its connection with the Doctrine of Signatures, which Porta elaborated upon (after Paracelsus) rather than created. The book has genuine scientific merit as well, for it groups plants ecologically by locale and distribution. (From Porta's *Phytognomonica*. Naples, H. Salviani, 1588. Original size 3 ¹/₁₆″ wide × 4 ¹/₈″ high.)

biosa, anything in fact that exhibited overlapping scales, could be employed in treating ailments characterized by scaly conditions of the skin. The kernels of walnuts, with their resemblance to the brain, and citrons, with a shape similar to the heart, relieved the ills of those organs. It was a far-fetched theory, but since it offered a simplified method of selecting appropriate remedies it quickly gained popular acceptance. Porta's *Phytognomonica* (Plant Indicators) was an elaborate exposition of its application. The notion was not entirely confined to medicine, but was applied to agriculture as well. In Porta's *Natural Magic* he advises the reader that the most certain way of raising larger gourds, cucumbers, or fruits was to choose seed from the widest part of the plant, or from its innermost and therefore richest parts.

This seemingly half-hearted attitude towards the natural sciences, wherein genuine truth was mingled with superstitions and false beliefs, was not unique to Porta. Alchemists, magicians, and prognosticators still held their ardent believers, and astrology was very much a part of pharmacy and medical practice. Tommaso Gianotti, called Rangoni, amassed a fortune in Venice by treating patients with herbal preparations gathered, compounded, and administered along astrological lines. He even published astrological calendars so that those unlearned in the art could choose or avoid lucky and unlucky days. A great flood was predicted in 1524 by the astrologer Stöffler, as a result of the conjunction of all the planets in Pisces. It turned out to be a year of drought, but even that inappropriate event did not disillusion the faithful, and astrology continued actively to invade the scientific realm in the 17th century. In 1649 an edition of Johannis Schröderi's *Medico-Chymica Pharmacopeia,* a respectable work on pharmacy, was published with an encyclopedic treatment of astrological methods meant to serve the apothecary. There were charts and tables that showed how to compute the changing positions of the planets, the hourly influences upon males and females, everything, in fact, necessary to the filling of prescriptions drawn up on astrological principles. Even as late as 1682, Abraham Munting, Doctor of Medicine and Professor of Botany at the Academy in Groeningen, deemed it necessary to publish information about the daily and hourly influences of the planets so that correct conditions for planting might be observed.

Porta, therefore, was very much in tune with his times, mingling strict logic and valid observations with practices more suited to soothsayers and magicians. Consider his advice on the soporific and mind-altering drug, mandragora:

> When you would use it, give it to somebody to drink; and whosoever shall taste it, after a deep sleep will be distracted and for a day shall rave: but after some sleep will return to his senses again, without any harm: and it is very pleasant to behold. Pray make trial.

Obviously medical advice had a way to go before it brought unequivocal benefit to man. And it may still be on the road to that goal.

BIBLIOGRAPHIC NOTES

1st edition: 1588 by Horatium Salvianum at Naples. Illustrated with 32 woodcuts.
2nd edition: 1591 by J. Wechel and P. Fischer at Frankfort.
3rd edition: 1608 by Nicklaus Hoffman at Frankfort.
4th edition: 1650 by I. Berthelin at Rothomagi (Rouen).

~§ 26 ξ~

The *Coloquios* of Garcia da Orta, and the *Dos Libros* of Nicolas Monardes

 HE 16th century was a time of exploration, when the European nations burst the confines of their small continent and sought out all the distant and unknown corners of the earth. Motivated by a mixture of curiosity and greed, kings, traders, and adventurers penetrated the fabled lands that Marco Polo had spoken of, and outdid his wildest tales with discovery of an Asiatic world that had long been unexplored. They journeyed about in what would now be considered mere cockleshells, many of them only thirty feet in length, and with superstructures that made them eminently capsizable in the tropical storms they encountered.

Much of their transoceanic shuttlings were focused on finding gold, gems, and expensive silks and spices, but they also added greatly to the world's store of knowledge about medicinal plants. All the mysterious substances that had filtered through to the west by way of Istanbul, Alexandria, and the bazaars of Syria and the Holy Land, could now be traced to their sources. And in addition to the drugs of the Orient was an untold wealth of other medicaments from the still untapped New World, many of which promised cures that bordered on the miraculous. Hearsay and legend were giving way at last to observation and examination as science began its own course of international exploration. The fantasies and inaccuracies of the herbals were soon to be replaced with precise botanical descriptions and the analytical methods of the chemists. The herbal still had its place, but it was entering its sunset years as factual reports about the world and its produce became accessible to men of learning. Two such accounts, both of prime importance, were the *Coloquios* of Garcia da Orta, on the *materia medica* of India, and the *Dos Libros* of Nicolas Monardes, about the drug substances of the West Indies and New Spain.

Born at Elvas near Badajos about 1490, Garcia da Orta was Portuguese, but received his medical education in Spain. Upon attaining his degree in 1525, after studies at Salamanca and Alcala de Henares, he became village physician at Castello de Vide in 1526. In 1532 he accepted a post as lecturer at the University of Lisbon, but two years later he sailed for the Portuguese colony of Goa. Either the journey or the destination cured da Orta's wanderlust, for he remained there as a practising physician until his death in 1570, some 36 years later.

During that time he had ample opportunity to investigate the medicinal plants and other materials of his adopted home, and his descriptions of them have had lasting value. Even as late as the 19th century his *Coloquios* were cited on seven occasions by Hanbury and Fluckiger in their monumental work, *Pharmacographia*. The *Coloquios* were the natural outgrowth of a lifetime spent in procuring as much knowledge as possible about the materials of medicine. In Europe, da Orta had amassed tremendous erudition concerning herbal literature, and could quote it at length. In

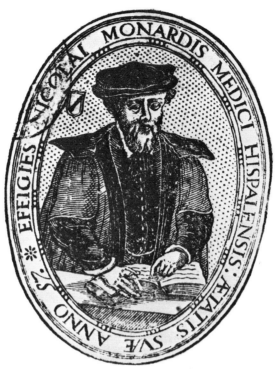

FIGURE 91. Portrait of Monardes. Nicolas Monardes was 57 years old when this portrait was done. Although he never visited the New World, he wrote knowledgeably about the medicinal properties of its drug-plants. He was also the author of treatises on the Bezoar Stone, the Herb Scorzonera, the refrigerant qualities of snow, and the medical uses of water containing iron. (From N. Monardes' *Dos Libros*. Seville, H. Dias, 1569. Original size 2 $^{11}/_{16}$" wide × 3 $^{5}/_{8}$" high.)

India he pursued a more direct course, questioning the native physicians, yogis, merchants, and travellers from every part of the Orient. Da Orta had also acquired the ability to read Avicenna in the original Arabic, and gathered plant names in a variety of tongues, including Persian, Hindu, and Malaysian. His descriptions of drug plants and their uses therefore gained an extra dimension because of his personal familiarity with them.

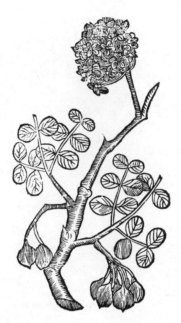

FIGURE 92. Guaiacum. According to Monardes, *Guaiacum officinale* is a sovereign remedy for the pox. In an account of how that undesirable disease first reached Europe, he attributes it to Indians from Santo Domingo who had been brought to Naples by Columbus in 1493 while peace was being celebrated by Naples and France. It was then called Spanish scab and Measles of the Indies. (From *Histoire des Drogues.* Lyon, J. Pillehotte, 1619. Original size 2 5/8" wide × 5" high.)

The *Coloquios* present da Orta's information in the form of 59 dialogues between himself and one Dr. Ruano, a fictitious alter ego who represented theoretical knowledge as opposed to the pragmatism of da Orta. Time and again da Orta replies "I have seen it" to Ruano's quotes from Dioscorides, Serapion, or Mattioli. He resolves questions about camphor, revealing it as an exudation from a tree, and perfectly white in its natural state, correcting the misconception that it was cleansed of black and vermilion streaks by washing or calci-

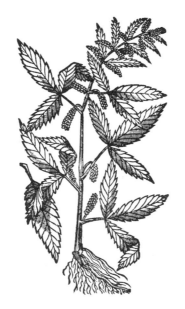

FIGURE 93. Bangue (Cannabis). Da Orta described the effects of bhang, *Cannabis sativa*,
in his eighth colloquy. There he speaks of its
use by women who want "to dally and flirt
with men," by those who wish to rise above
care, and others who seek rest and sleep.
The Sultan Bahadur is quoted in regard to its
hallucinogenic action saying that "he had
only to take bhang when he wished to journey about the world at night." (From *Histoire
des Drogues* . . . Lyon, J. Pillehotte, 1619.
Original size 2 ¹/₂" wide × 4 ³/₄" high.)

nation. And da Orta made his readers aware that cloves and
nutmegs came from entirely different trees, despite tales that
they were the flower and the fruit of one and the same plant.

In the conversations with Dr. Ruano there are many
sensible statements about aloes, cannabis, styrax, coconut,
rauwolfia, lacquer, ginger, and other produce of the Orient.
In the *Coloquios,* da Orta departs widely from the standard
format of the herbal, the end result being an integrated study
of sources, techniques, economics, customs, manners, and
ethnology. He never restricts himself entirely to medicine,

but brings in such topics as the taming of elephants, the production of cinnamon, the Indian names of chessmen, Indian fables, and travels to the Spice Islands. Now and then he falls into error, as when he says white and black pepper are two separate kinds, but he was misled by those who raised the vine. The fact was that they could prepare the white sort, which sold for an exorbitant price, simply by removing the thin outer cortex before grinding the peppercorns into powder.

The *Coloquios* was first printed in Goa in 1563, the third book ever to be printed in India, and it is extremely rare. A second edition, of equal rarity, was also published at Goa, but neither were well known to 16th-century Europeans. Both were in da Orta's Portuguese. In Europe, knowledge of the work came about through the Latin translation and abridgement made by Charles de l'Escluse (Clusius) for a publication issued by the Plantin press of Antwerp in 1567. Italian and French translations were made from the Latin edition but, like the Latin edition, they bear little resemblance to the original. Another edition in Portuguese was done at Lisbon in 1872, but it is replete with gaps and other imperfections. Not until 1891, when the Conde de Ficalho brought out an annotated edition of da Orta's work, was it truly available to the botanical and pharmaceutical worlds, which had previously known it largely from the abridged form made by Clusius. Despite the fact that it had waited over three hundred years to gain recognition, the *Coloquios* still had much to offer.

The *Dos Libros* of Nicolas Monardes served the European community by publicizing many of the new drug plants from America, but it is something less than a model of accuracy. Monardes, who was born about 1493 in Seville and practiced there after taking his medical degree at the University of Alcala de Henares, never visited the New World, and so was an imperfect judge not only of its sub-

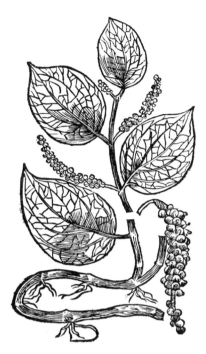

FIGURE 94. Pepper. Europeans thought pepper came from a tree, but it was actually the product of a climbing vine. The black variety came from peppercorns that retained their husks, while the considerably more expensive white kind was made from decorticated seeds. The fiction of the rare white pepper, fit for royalty only at royal prices, was maintained for several centuries. The Western mind was sometimes a bit laggard in seeing the truth. (From *Histoire des Drogues* . . . Lyon, J. Pillehotte, 1619. Original size 2 ³/₄″ wide × 5 ³/₁₆″ high.)

stances that Spain imported but also of the tales that accompanied them. Monardes, however, was not the questioning sort, and welcomed the wonders that were told to him. He speaks of a wood that, although white itself, turned water clear blue and transformed it into an effective cure for stones in the kidneys or the bladder. It also healed obstructions of

the spleen and ailments of the lungs and liver. Then there
was Mechoacan, an even greater panacea, that cured dropsy,
jaundice, scrofula, migraine, gout, colic, rheumatism, fevers, epilepsy, chest and lung conditions, and the pox (by
which Monardes meant syphilis). Cures also resulted from
use of the Bezoar stone, a concretion found in the internal
organs of animals. The good doctor even credited it with
healing a case of leprosy.

Along with the nonsense went descriptions of such important plants as tobacco (one of the first pictures of it was
in Monardes' book), and coca, a stimulant and anodyne that
was to have great consequence for anesthetists and illegal
drug dealers. There is also mention of the sunflower, pas-
sion-flower, guava, sarsaparilla, and balsam, but nothing is
said of quinine, which had to wait almost another century to
be discovered.

Monardes apparently lived a quiet life in Seville. Little is recorded other than his death in 1578. Besides his
famous *Dos Libros,* to which a third part was added posthumously, he wrote a few other medical tracts, among them
three which are commonly appended to his major work:
"On the Bezoar Stone and the Herb Scorzonera (Viper-
grass)," "The Dialogue on Iron," and "Of the Snow and the
Virtues Thereof." There is little doubt that Frampton's translation of the *Dos Libros,* which transformed it into the ebul-
lient *Joyfull Newes Out of the Newe Founde Worlde,* gave the
good doctor greater repute than was his due, for nowhere
does Monardes approach da Orta in verity and exactitude.
Aside from the value inherent in any early report of things
newly discovered, the greatest merit in Monardes is his
pleasantly discursive style, with its naive delight in marvels
and wonders.

BIBLIOGRAPHIC NOTES

Garcia da Orta (sometimes listed as ab Horto or del Huerto). *Coloquios dos simples, e drogas he cousas mediçinais da India.*

1st edition: 1563 by Joannes de Endem at Goa. In Portuguese. A second Portuguese edition, also at Goa, is reported by Markham, without naming either date or printer. Pritzel does not mention it.

1st Latin edition: 1567 by Carolo Clusio for Christophori Plantini at Antwerp. Further editions of this digest of da Orta were issued by the Plantin press in 1574, 1579, 1593, and 1605, the last being part of Clusius' *Exoticorum libri decem.*

1st English edition: 1577 at London, printer and translator not given by Pritzel. Translated from the Latin of Clusius.

1st Italian edition: 1582 by Annibal Briganti, printed at Venice. Printer not given by Pritzel.

1st French edition: 1619 (Pritzel says 2nd edition) by Antoine Colin at Lyons for the printer, Pillehotte.

19th-century printings of Portuguese text:
1872 by F. A. de Varnhagen at Lisbon. Poorly edited.
1891, the standard version, edited by the Conde de Ficalho, at Lisbon. Printer not named by Markham.

1st English translation of Ficalho's edition: 1913 by Sir Clements R. Markham, for Henry Sotheran and Co., London.

Nicolas Monardes. *Dos libros, el uno que trata de todas las cosas que traen de nuestras Indias Occidentales.*

1st edition: 1569 by Hernando Diaz at Seville.
2nd edition: 1571 by Alonso Escrivano at Seville.
3rd edition: 1574 at Seville, printer not given by Pritzel or Arber.
4th edition: 1580 by Fernando Diaz at Seville.
1st Latin edition: 1574 by Christophori Plantini at Antwerp. Trans. from the original Spanish by Clusius. Others in 1579 and 1582.
1st English edition: 1577 by Jhon Frampton, printed by W. Norton at London. Title, *Joyfull Newes Out of the Newe Founde Worlde.*

~§ 27 §~

The *Phytobasanos* of Fabio Colonna

HE odd-sounding title of Fabio Colonna's first botanical publication, *Phytobasanos*, simply means "plant touchstone." Touchstones were marble slabs used by goldsmiths to determine a metal's value and quality. One merely drew the metal across the surface and judged it by the colored streak it left. Colonna's book was intended to be a touchstone for plants by providing a positive means of identification. It was a rather ambitious project for a young man of 25, and at a time when botany could scarcely be called a science. Yet, thanks to Colonna's efforts and those of other Renaissance inquirers, the study of plants was moving ever nearer to becoming a science.

Born in Naples in 1567, Colonna was a member of an illustrious family that could trace its history back to the days of the Roman Empire. Soldiers, poets, and prelates were numbered among his relations, for the Colonnas always managed somehow to be in the forefront of affairs in Italy. Fabio had been raised with all the advantages of wealth, including access to his father's extensive library of some 2,500 volumes, a sizable collection for the time. Educated as a lawyer, Colonna also pursued a variety of other interests, and was more than passingly adept in mathematics, languages, music, optics, drawing, and botany. He was, in short, a perfect example of the Renaissance man, one of those extraordinarily inquisitive minds who followed the torch of learning wherever it led, and did so for enjoyment as much as for knowledge.

Unfortunately, though, Colonna's good fortune was balanced by some bad, for he was burdened throughout his life by epilepsy. He was troubled by it from adolescence, but rather than suffer in quiet resignation, he actively sought out means of relief. Since medicine at that time was based almost entirely on plant products, it was only natural that Colonna turned to a systematic investigation of medicinal plants. Thanks to his tireless and pains-taking efforts, he finally discovered a useful remedy in the root of *Valeriana officinalis,* which contains an ingredient that has a sedative effect upon the higher nerve centers and is also an anticonvulsant. Unfortunately it loses effectiveness after continued use, a fact with which Colonna eventually had to contend.

Incidentally, it is sometimes said that Colonna was seeking out the kind of valerian that Dioscorides had prescribed for epilepsy, but this is pure legend. Dioscorides was ignorant of its use for that disease. The myth seems to have begun in the early 19th century in Rees's *Cyclopedia,* which claims that Albrecht von Haller made a statement to that effect. But since it is known that von Haller read Greek, it is not likely that he would have mistaken Dioscorides' text. Colonna himself, then, must be regarded as the first to use valerian as a specific for epilepsy.

In his studies leading to the discovery of valerian as an alleviator of his illness, Colonna found a lack of concordance in the descriptions of plants. Having combed the works of

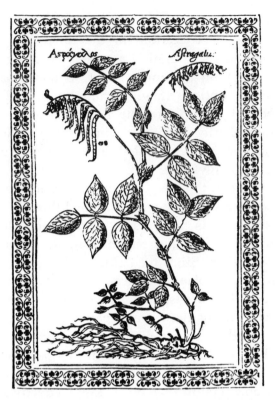

FIGURE 95. Astragalus. Although it is of the *Leguminosae* family, this plant is not an Astragalus as that genus is currently classified. In regard to the printing technique: the border of the picture is printed from the raised surface of a woodcut, the plant from lines etched down into a copper plate. Paper, therefore, had to pass through the press twice to receive impressions from the two opposed elements, and a means of preventing overlap had to be devised to keep the two images in register. This seems to be the earliest attempt to use the technique on a single side of a sheet. (From Colonna's *Phytobasanos*. Naples, H. Salviani, 1592. Original size 4" wide × 6 1/16" high.)

Theophrastus, Hippocrates, Pliny, Galen, Dioscorides, and others for a remedy, he was keenly aware of the need to bring more order into writings on *materia medica* and botany. He was also aware of the great value of accurate pictures that clearly showed the unique characteristics of indi-

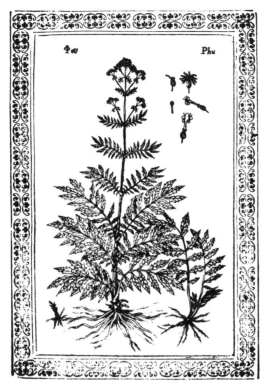

FIGURE 96. Phu. In the course of Colonna's search for the true identity of this plant, which Dioscorides had called Phu, he became a botanist. The plant is Great Wild Valerian, which was used by the ancients as an aromatic and a diuretic, but Colonna employed it successfully upon himself as an antispasmodic for epileptic seizures. The effect, however, lessened with continued use. (From Colonna's *Phytobasanos*. Naples, H. Salviani, 1592. Original size 4 ¹/₁₆" wide × 6" high.)

vidual plants. He thus constructed his *Phytobasanos* with these aims in mind.

Since he was skilled in drawing, Colonna drew his chosen plant specimens himself. To reproduce them, he chose etching, a means new to botanical book-illustration. The sharp but delicate lines produced by the etching needle preserved a wealth of details that were inevitably lost by the

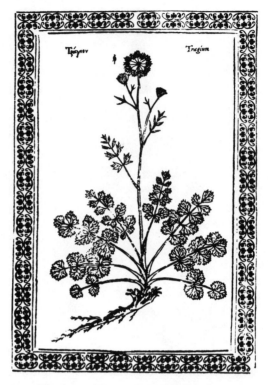

FIGURE 97. Tragium (Goat's Beard). The plant that Colonna called Tragium was later called the Greater Burnet
Saxifrage. It was so named not because it was either Burnet
or Saxifrage, but because it had leaves like Burnet and
was thought to break up stones in the bladder (Saxifrage
means stone-breaker in Latin). Such loose nomenclature
was typical of pre-Linnaean botany. The plant is now
known as *Pimpinella magna*. (From Colonna's *Phytobasanos*. Naples, H. Salviani, 1592. Original size 4 $^{1}/_{16}$"
wide × 6" high.)

heavier lines of woodcuts, but they also introduced a problem. Etched designs are bitten down into the surface of a
plate, while type is raised above the surface. Type and
etched plates, therefore, could not be printed at the same
time on the same press. Colonna solved the difficulty, not as
more timid publishers did later on by putting the illustrations on separate sheets that followed the body of the text,

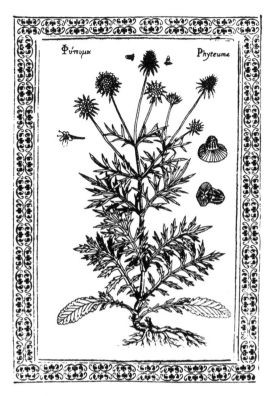

FIGURE 98. Phyteuma. In modern botany the name *Phyteuma* refers to a genus in the Bellflower family, the *Campanulaceae*. Here, however, Colonna is concerned with one of the Scabious group, very likely Field Scabious, a plant that was credited with a variety of virtues. It dissolved carbuncles, restored shrunken veins and sinews, healed wounds, sores, and ulcers, and cured pleurisy, leprosy, and even dandruff. (From Colonna's *Phytobasanos*. Naples, H. Salviani, 1592. Original size 4″ wide × 6″ high.)

but by running the sheets through the press a second time. That meant that the designs had to land exactly on the blank space reserved for them, in this case within a printed border. Colonna thus produced one of the earliest examples in printing of multiple register on a single page side. Two novel techniques within the covers of one book, plus a cure new to medicine—quite an accomplishment for a 25-year-old beginner.

It is little wonder that Colonna was called upon to help organize the Accademia dei Lincei, which included Galileo and himself as charter members. During his long years of association with that scientific society he invented a complicated 50-stringed instrument (the sambuca Lyncia), helped edit an invaluable publication on the New World (the *Thesaurus Rerum Medicarum* of Francisco Hernandez), and continued his study of botany. He was the first to add the word "petal" to the botanists' vocabulary, and contributed to the concept of genera. Later botanists such as Thomas Johnson, reviser of Gerard's *Herball*, Carl Linnaeus, and Michel Adanson praised Colonna's exactitude and judgment. Writing at a time when the sexuality of plants was still unknown, he had this to say about setting up a system of classification:

> I do not value the shape of the leaf in making up the Genera of Plants, but I determine their kindred and family to which they belong by the flower and seed vessels, or rather the seed itself, especially if they agree by the taste with the other parts of the plant. This is what has not been observed by botanists before this time, neither by Dioscorides himself nor yet by the ancients.

Later he clearly stated that plants could be differentiated by their stamens and styles, plainly indicating the path that Linnaeus would follow. Colonna's two major botanical works, the *Phytobasanos* and its sequel the *Ekphrasis* (Exposition), were valuable contributions that led to the concepts of genera and species. Both books contain skilfully executed plates that set new standards for botanical illustration, and rely almost entirely on line for their effect, using only minimal shading.

Although largely concerned with herbs and *materia medica*, Colonna's emphasis was not primarily on their medicinal uses, but was botanical instead. He sought to identify precisely the plants described by Dioscorides and other classical writers, but much of his aim was frustrated by those writers' terms, their likening of parts of some plants to parts of others, and the very broad standards of their classifications.

Colonna had advanced the cause of biology as well as botany, and replaced fantasies with reality. For example, he was among the first to demonstrate that the tale of the Barnacle Goose, supposedly generated from barnacle-laden timbers, was purely imaginary. His etching of barnacles, the marine organisms that provided the base for the story, was as accurate and esthetic as any of his botanical works had been.

After a lifetime of repeated epileptic attacks, Colonna's faculties finally failed, and he died in 1651 at the age of 83. He had always believed that the wonders of nature were greater than those of fable, and his *Phytobasanos* is a testament to that belief.

BIBLIOGRAPHIC NOTES

1st edition: 1592 by J. J. Carlinum at Naples, with 38 etched plates set in letter-press borders. The etchings are by Colonna himself. The original drawings were rediscovered in the 19th century in the Biblioteca Nazionale in Naples.

2nd edition: 1744 by Viviani at Florence. This contains a life of Colonna by Iano Planco written in Latin. Copies of the original plates were printed for the edition but are set after the text and lack the ornamental letter-press borders.

◦⟨ 28 ⟩◦

The *Herball* of John Gerard

ERARD'S *Herball*, if not one of the monu-
ments of the English language, is certainly
one of its great delights. Despite the passage
of time, which has long since outmoded his
medical recommendations, Gerard continues to be in strong
demand. It is entirely possible, in fact, that copies of Gerard
printed in the 20th century far outnumber those printed in
the 16th and 17th centuries. The Herball's popularity is
beyond question, but Gerard's share in its creation is not, as
we will see later.

Born at Nantwich, Cheshire, in 1545, Gerard was
schooled at Wisterson, now Willaston, and in 1562 was ap-
prenticed to Alexander Mason, a Warden of the Barber-
Surgeons' Company. About this time he travelled, probably
as a ship's surgeon, along the Baltic coast. Little is known of
his family background, since his baptismal record was lost
along with many others at Nantwich, but his coat of arms
assigns him to a branch of the Gerards of Ince in Lancashire.
The College of Arms, however, holds no information about
his parentage. It is possible that he was of more consequential lineage than the facts display. There is no doubt that

when he came to London he soon made influential friends and apparently enjoyed an ample income, since he owned a house in Holborn, then a rich and aristocratic neighborhood.

Gerard became the superintendent of the gardens of William Cecil, Lord Burghley, one of the most powerful figures at the court of Elizabeth I. The gardens were located in the Strand in London, and at Theobalds in Hertfordshire. Gerard also had an extensive garden of his own in Holborn where he raised not only the native plants of England, but numerous exotic ones sent to him from overseas. His picture of the potato, probably the earliest known, and his description of it were an outgrowth of his connections with Raleigh, Drake, and the colonizers of the New World. A potato plant was supplied to him for his garden long before it became a common item.

The precise year that he arrived in London is not known, but it must have been before February 21, 1577. He was issued a summons on that date by the Master of the Barber-Surgeons' Company on a charge of defaming the wife of another member. At a much later date, October 1606, Gerard was fined for abusing John Peck, an Examiner of the Company. But two such isolated instances are not sufficient evidence for assuming he was contentious, any more than they are for assuming he was meek and mild.

Although Gerard would seem to have been fully occupied with the care of three gardens, he still found time to be actively engaged in the affairs of the Barber-Surgeons' Company, which was then a very powerful body in control of the practice of surgery. Gerard was quite proud of his association with it since he included its coat of arms with his own as embellishments to his portrait in the *Herball*. He became a junior warden of the Company in 1597 and an Examiner in 1598. Then he moved to Second Warden and Upper Governor. He resigned from the latter office in September 1605, but by August 1608 he was elected Master of

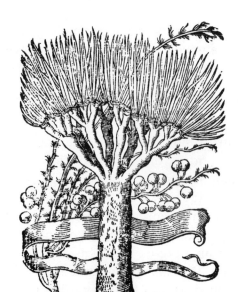

FIGURE 99. Dragon Tree. A native of the Canary Islands, the Dragon Tree is the true source of the reddish resin known as dragon's blood. The tree, which is related to asparagus, reaches a great size and age. Alexander von Humboldt spoke of one at Orotava that was 70 feet high and had a diameter of 15 feet. It was estimated to be several thousand years old. (From Gerard's *Herball*. London, J. Norton, 1597. Original size 3" wide × 5 ¼" high.)

the Company. He died in 1612 and was buried in St. Andrew's Church, Holborn, but the burial plot is unmarked. Vital records concerning his life consistently disappeared; even the records of the Barber-Surgeons' Company during his term as Master have vanished.

The facts surrounding Gerard's participation in the *Herball* are equally clouded and inconclusive, despite the fact that the work bears his name. He seems to have been called upon to aid John Norton, the Queen's printer, when a difficulty arose. Norton had engaged a certain Dr. Priest to do a

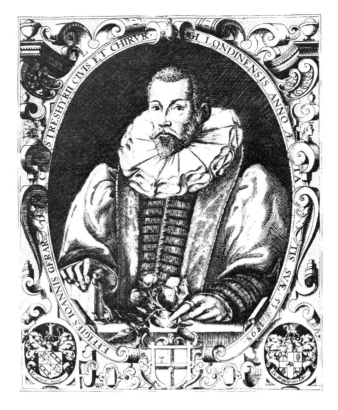

FIGURE 100. Portrait of Gerard. John Gerard, native of Chester and member of the Barber-Surgeon's Company of London, is shown here at the age of 53. Although the engraved portrait bears the date 1598, it appeared in the first edition of Gerard's *Herball*, published in 1597. The flower he is holding is that of the potato, a plant pictured for the first time in this book. (From Gerard's *Herball*. London, J. Norton, 1597. Original size 5 ⁵⁄₈" wide × 7" high.)

new translation of Rembert Dodoens' *Pemptades*, then a highly regarded herbal, and one well known in England through Henry Lyte's translation. Priest died before the translation was fully ready for the press, and Norton needed someone with a knowledge of plants to bring the venture to a successful close. Somehow Gerard's name came to his notice, perhaps through mutual acquaintances at the Royal Court, or through Gerard's reputation as a horticulturist, or

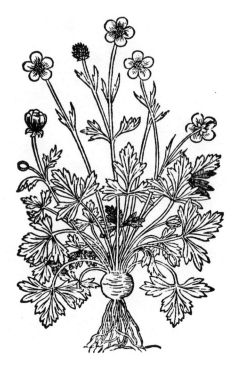

FIGURE 101. Round-rooted Crowfoot. Gerard's Round-rooted Crowfoot is a member of the Buttercup family, the *Ranunculaceae,* its modern scientific name being *Ranunculus bulbosus.* Gerard mentions the use by beggars of its acrid, blistering properties. They applied the crushed leaves to their arms and legs so as to create ulcers and thus gain sympathy. The uncertain, poisonous action of Crowfoot made it dangerous in remedies. (From Gerard's *Herball.* London, J. Norton, 1597. Original size 3″ wide × 5 ¼″ high.)

with the publication in 1596 of a catalogue to Gerard's own garden. The catalogue was the first work of its kind, a complete inventory of a private garden listing some 1,039 plants, so Norton had good reason to select Gerard for his project.

For a while Gerard simply did what he was asked, but then he took a different turn. Priest had been making a translation of Dodoens, but Gerard argued that since Priest was dead, his work had perished with him. Gerard there-

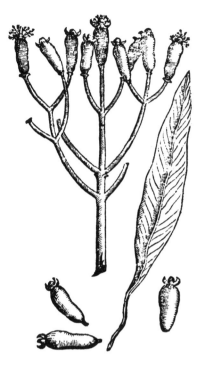

FIGURE 102. Cloves. Gerard stated that cloves were hot and dry in the third degree. They were gathered from September to February, not by picking but by beating the tree, as was done in England with walnuts. He also said that four drams of powdered cloves taken in milk "procureth the act of generation." (From Gerard's *Herball*. London, J. Norton, 1597. Original size 2 5/8" wide × 5 3/8" high.)

upon changed the arrangement of the book to the system of another botanist, L'Obel, rather than that of Dodoens, probably hoping to pass it off as a new work rather than simply a new translation. Perhaps Norton urged such a course, perhaps not, but the result was obvious plagiarism. A comparison of Lyte's translation with associated passages in Gerard makes the source of the *Herball* all too evident.

Gerard, however, was in over his head, for there were many plants in the *Herball* that were unknown to him, and

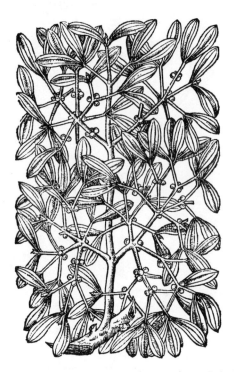

FIGURE 103. Mistletoe. Gathered from oaks in Britain since the days of the Druids, Mistletoe was regarded by Gerard as the best material for birdlime, but he describes no other uses for it. It has been used, however, to treat epilepsy, given in small dosages. Large doses induce the opposite effect, causing convulsions. The sticky birdlime was also applied to sores and ulcers. (From Gerard's *Herball*. London, J. Norton, 1597. Original size 3" wide × 5 ¼" high.)

he had the onerous task of matching their descriptions to the proper woodcuts. These were rented by Norton from the Frankfort publisher of Tabernaemontanus' herbal. L'Obel, the Flemish botanist, finally had to be called in to straighten out the tangle, and made over 1,000 corrections. Gerard, however, became impatient with L'Obel's rate of progress and cut the work short. The *Herball* then went to press, errors and all.

It is a complicated story, and one that leaves doubt as to

who should be credited with what in the total production of
the *Herball.* Perhaps it would be best to call it an uncon-
scious collaboration. There are the botanical contributions of
Dodoens and L'Obel, both fully documented, and the translations of both Lyte and Priest. There is also the fact that
L'Obel's English, faulty as it may have been, made up for
the deficiencies of Gerard's Latin. The remainder (and that
is the appropriate word), which consists of the highlighting
of indigenous plants, locations cited for English flora (some
of them spurious), mention of specific personalities, and
other topical matter that gave the book its unique flavor, are
very likely all of Gerard's own doing. But he suffered a severe case of ague from 1596 to 1599 that was damaging
enough to delay preparation of the second edition of his catalogue, so where did he find the energy to edit and rewrite
some 1,392 pages of text? The time might actually have been
available to him though, for London had then experienced
such bad weather for several years that almost nothing
grew. The grain crops were down to famine level, and wheat
sold for five pounds four shillings a quarter (eight bushels),
a price equivalent in purchasing power to almost 150 current
dollars.

Gerard's *Herball,* in all honesty, should be recognized as
Dodoens' *Herbal* with English dress, manners, and substance. In a sense Gerard did much the same with Dodoens
as Shakespeare had done with the tales of Boccaccio or Ho-
linshed's *Chronicles,* save that Gerard was not offering fiction, which does make a difference. The pity is that he need
not have gone to such pains to hide what was evident to
anyone who could read, for his contemporaries and poster-
ity both loaded the book with praises. The well-written
words of Lyte's version, which Priest may in turn have bet-
tered, took on a vivifying glow under Gerard's touch. His
expertise as a surgeon may be debatable, but his expertise
with language was not. He may have been a scoundrel, like
the cut-purse François Villon, but his words were pure gold.

Who could deny the charm of such names as "Clown's Woundwort" and "Traveller's Joy"? His description of dandelion heads is pure poetry: "a floure . . . thick set together, of colour yellow, which is turned into a round downy blowbal that is carried away with the wind." His commendation of Eye-bright says that it "taketh away all hurts from the eyes, comforteth the memorie, and cleareth the sight. . . ." And a passage on violets states: "for that very many by these violets receive ornament and comely grace . . . and the recreation of the minde which is taken hereby cannot be but very good and honest . . . for floures through their beauty . . . do bring to a liberall and gentle manly minde the remembrance of . . . all kindes of virtues. . . ." The man who wrote that deserves forgiveness for the one moment that *he* lost his comely grace and remembrance of virtue.

BIBLIOGRAPHIC NOTES

1st edition: 1597 by John Norton at London. 1,800 woodcuts, first
     used to illustrate the 1590 edition of Tabernaemontanus. 16
     were original, including the picture of the potato.
2nd edition: 1633, edited by Thomas Johnson, who enlarged and
     corrected it, published by Norton and Whitakers, at London.
     2,821 woodcuts.
3rd edition: 1636, other data same as above.

◄§ 29 §►

Parkinson's *Theatrum Botanicum*

 H E title page of the *Theater of Plants,* to use its English name, proclaims it as "An Herball of Large Extent." It is, for there are 1,755 folio sized pages, over 2,700 woodcuts, and the descriptions of more than 3,800 plants. If a reader should happen to drop it on his foot he would be well advised to consult the passages on comfrey or other plants good for mending broken bones. Considered to be the last of the great herbals, the *Theatrum Botanicum* lives up to its reputation, in size as well as in quality.

The author of the work, John Parkinson, was born in Nottinghamshire in 1567. There is no further record of him until 1616, when he had become a practicing apothecary with a garden of his own in Long Acre, now almost the center of London. Parkinson was first appointed Apothecary to James I, and later in 1629 Charles I honored him with the title, "Botanicus Regius Primarius." He was well acquainted with the editor and reviser of Gerard's *Herball,* Thomas Johnson, and with the owner of a famous museum in Lambeth, John Tradescant. His was a quiet but industrious life, devoted to gardening and the study of medicinal plants. In

227

1650 he died, and was buried in the Church of St. Martin's-in-the-Fields, adjoining what is now Trafalgar Square.

Parkinson is probably better known for his *Paradisi in Sole Paradisus Terrestris* than for his herbal. The title of this first work was actually a pun on his own name, for the Latin words translate into "Park in sun's earthly paradise." The book was dedicated to Queen Henrietta Maria, and Parkinson termed it a "feminine work of flowers." Its emphasis was purely horticultural, since by his time the interest in ornamental planting had increased greatly, and gardens were no longer almost exclusively devoted to the uses of the kitchen and the still room. Parkinson pictured and described "all sorts of pleasant flowers which our English ayre will permitt to be noursed up." He inferred that each garden was, or could be, a little Eden of its own. To underscore the point, the title page showed Adam and Eve strolling through the glades of Paradise.

The work included 109 woodcuts of some 780 plants. Unluckily the cuts were somewhat clumsy in style, and no match for Parkinson's text, which had an Elizabethan grace, color, and vigor. The shortcomings of the pictures do not seem to have handicapped the work, however, since it was reprinted in 1656 and again in 1904.

The *Theatrum Botanicum*, his second and major work, was as diplomatically dedicated as his first, this time to Charles I, and was called a "Manlike Worke of Herbes and Plants." In it Parkinson borrowed from the whole range of writings on *materia medica*, adding his own considerable knowledge as horticulturist and apothecary, to produce one of the great repositories of herbal literature. His references to older authors and his quotations from them make the *Theatrum* a virtual one-volume herbal library. Should all other herbals be lost, future generations could still sample most of their lore and language through Parkinson.

Although he lived in Jacobean and Carolean times there was also a distinctly medieval tone to Parkinson's thinking.

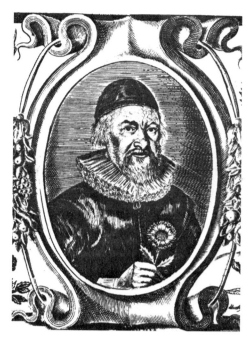

FIGURE 104. Portrait of Parkinson. John Parkinson's portrait for the *Theatrum Botanicum* of 1640 shows him in his latter years, aged a little over 70. He looks every inch the bluff and forthright English gardener that his text reveals him to be. The flower he holds is one of the Compositae family, but the species is uncertain. (From Parkinson's *Theatrum Botanicum*. London, T. Cotes, 1640. Original size 2″ wide × 2 ⅝″ high.)

He accepted the existence of the unicorn, although he located it in regions as remote from man's habitation as it was from factuality. He also continued the legend of the Vegetable Lamb, a plant said to carry a small, wool-bearing lamb at the head of its stalk. It browsed on herbage that grew nearby, and when that was gone it died, unless the wolves devoured it first. The origin of the tale was the Asiatic cotton plant, which produced a substance many people took to be a finer, softer kind of wool.

In Parkinson's time each of the plant sciences was beginning to define its own domain. Even Parkinson's *Para-*

disus *Terrestris* is claimed to be the first book that "separately described and figured the subjects of the flower garden." *Materia medica* was also being placed in its own category, and the same could be said for agriculture and silviculture. Botany was even being granted an independent position which recognized that systematic knowledge of the relationships and characteristics of plants was fully equal in importance to understanding their specific uses. Parkinson himself was aware of these shifts in emphasis, for in a foreword to the reader he says, "And although by the revolution of time it hath changed the note (that is from a Physicall Garden of Simples, to a Theater of Plants) yet not the nature, yea rather it hath gained the more matter by the overture. . . ."

Whether or not he realized that he was creating the last of its kind, Parkinson ploughed valiantly ahead in the production of his colossus among herbals. He still arranged plants with reference to their properties rather than to their natural affinities, dividing the plant world into seventeen tribes. Parkinson's first tribe bore the title "Sweet Smelling Herbes," in which he placed such unrelated plants as hyssop, thyme, parasitic dodder, marjoram, and polium. It was a poor system at best, ignoring obvious differences while favoring one common trait. His second tribe was mostly purgative plants, his third "Venemous, Sleepy and Hurtfull" ones, while his seventeenth was "Strange and Outlandish Plants," where the Vegetable Lamb must certainly have felt at home.

FIGURE 105. Title page of *Theatrum Botanicum*. Parkinson's *Theatre of Plants* opened with a magnificent allegorical title page that depicted signs of divine guidance: "a cloud by day, a pillar of fire by night," and the presence of Adam, the first gardener, and Solomon, wisest of men. They were intended as a guarantee of the contents, and the scope of the work was well indicated by showing plants from the various continents. (From Parkinson's *Theatrum Botanicum*. London, T. Cotes, 1640. Reduced from original size, 7 1/2" wide × 12 1/2" high.)

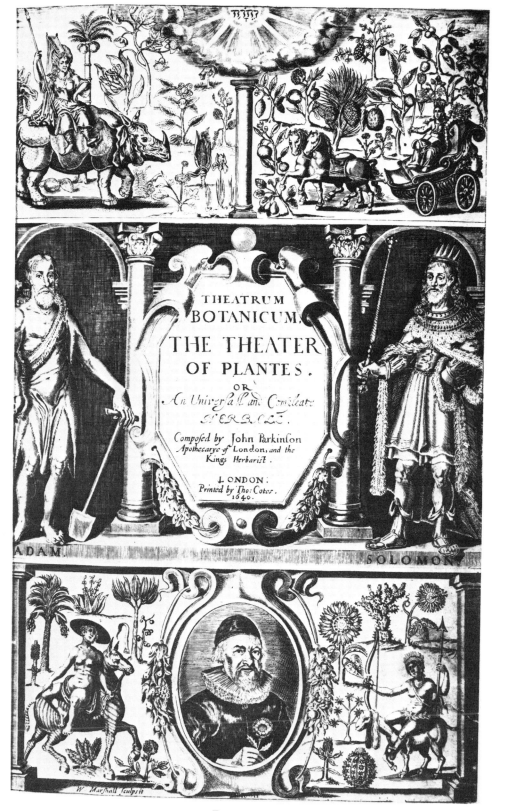

FIGURE 105.

Despite the quirks acquired from his training and his era, Parkinson was able to make some improvements in the herbal literature that was handed down to him. Like Isidore of Seville he seemed to have faith that knowledge of a thing's name conferred proper knowledge of the thing itself. In the *Paradisus* Parkinson has this to say about the creation of Adam:

> For, as he was able to give names to all the living Creatures, according to their severall natures; so no doubt but hee had also the knowledge, both what Herbes and Fruits were fit eyther for Meate or Medicine, for Use or for Delight.

This being a tenet of Parkinson's faith, he diligently sought out as complete a list of names and synonyms as possible, correcting errors that had multiplied through the centuries. Luckily for him, Caspar Bauhin in 1623 had compiled a monumental study on that subject, the *Phytopinax* (Table of Plants), and Parkinson put it to advantageous use in the *Theatrum* for the benefit of English gardeners and apothecaries.

The amplification and correction of nomenclature were not Parkinson's only contributions. He introduced 7 new plants into England, and was responsible for the first mention of some 33 different native plants. Thirteen of those were part of the Middlesex flora, in the London area, and had gone unnoticed by such illustrious predecessors as William Turner, John Goodyer, the famous (or infamous)

FIGURE 106. Title page of *Paradisi in Sole*. Parkinson's earlier book, the *Paradisi in Sole*, had a title page every bit as interesting as the later *Theatrum Botanicum*. Adam and Eve are seen wandering through the glades of Eden, enjoying pineapples, date palms, grape vines, and all the joys of peace and plenty. The Vegetable Lamb, apparently a favorite of Parkinson's, is figured near the apple tree close to the center of Paradise. (From Parkinson's *Paradisi in Sole* . . . London, Lownes and Young, 1629. Reduced from original size, 7 1/2" wide × 12 3/8" high.)

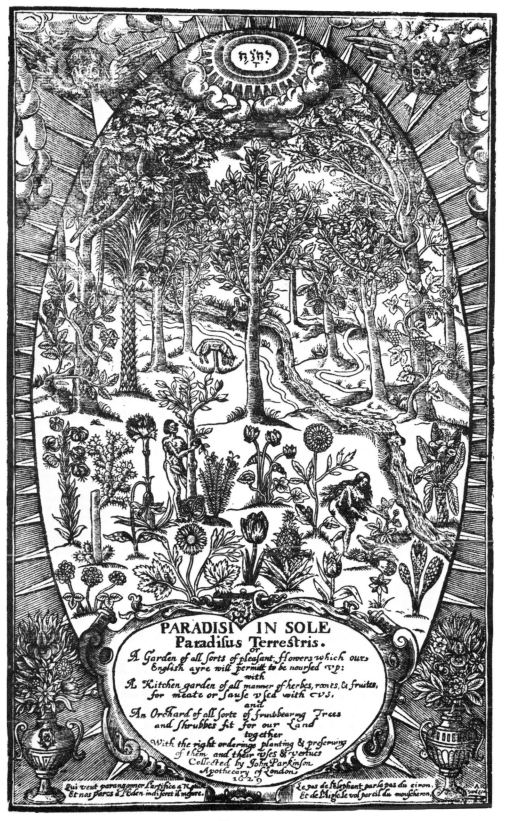

PARADISI IN SOLE
Paradiſus Terreſtris.
Or
A Garden of all ſorts of pleaſant flowers which our
Engliſh ayre will permitt to be noursed vp:
with
A Kitchen garden of all manner of herbes, rootes, & fruites,
for meate or ſauſe vſed with vs.
and
An Orchard of all ſorte of frubbearing Trees
and ſhrubbes fit for our Land
together
With the right orderinge planting & preſeruing
of them and their vſes & vertues
Collected by Iohn Parkinson
Apothecary of London.
1629

Qui veut parangonner l'artifice a l'art,   Le pas de l'elephant par le pas du ciron,
Et nos parcs à l'Eden, meſ ſoret il meſure.   Et de l'Aigle le vol par cil du mouſcheron.

FIGURE 106.

Gerard, and such perceptive plantsmen as Thomas Johnson and John Tradescant in Parkinson's own time. One wonders about the sharpness of human observation, for three of Parkinson's English "firsts" were such conspicuous plants as the Welsh Poppy, the Strawberry Tree, and Lady's Slipper.

The *Theatrum* was not the first herbal to knowingly incorporate plants that had no discernible economic or medicinal use, but it included far more of them than any herbal that had gone before. The old order was passing, and the new one, though still imperfectly understood, was waiting in the wings. John Ray, whose work helped turn the gropings of 16th- and 17th-century naturalists into the orderly methods of science, quoted extensively from the *Theatrum* and the *Paradisus,* and Parkinson's own intelligent contemporaries, such as Goodyer, Johnson, and Tradescant, held him in high regard.

Herbals, of course, continued to be compiled and reprinted, but their time had passed. Nothing new was added by any subsequent production, nor did any of them equal Parkinson in scope. The *Theatrum* marked a glorious sunset on the age of herbals, and it left a glow that will last as long as the English language is read.

BIBLIOGRAPHIC NOTES

1st edition: 1640 by Thomas Cotes at London.

No other editions published. A fragment, 24 pages, of the *Theatrum* was reprinted by the Herb Grower Press of Falls Village, Connecticut, no date, but about 1970.

◄§ 30 ◊►

The *Rerum Medicarum* of
Francisco Hernandez

 VEN as "the best-laid schemes o' mice and men gang aft agley," so do those of kings and medicos. A classic instance is that of an inventory requested by Philip II concerning the natural history of New Spain, which we now call Mexico. The task was entrusted to Dr. Francisco Hernandez, Philip's chamber physician at the Escorial, who was also charged with reporting on the antiquities and the political conditions of the region. That assignment may have roused a certain amount of hostility in New Spain, for Hernandez encountered a notable lack of cooperation there from local officials who were supposed to aid him in his endeavors. However, it is also possible that Hernandez himself, who seems to have been obsessed with the importance of his mission, may have brought about some of the hostility through demands that he made.

Relatively little is known of Hernandez himself. Even the date of his birth is uncertain, although it is estimated to be about 1514. His place of birth is not known either. Some

Spanish authorities say it was Seville, while the majority say Toledo. What is certain is that he attended the University of Salamanca, graduated from there, and joined its faculty. Eventually Hernandez came to the attention of Philip II and entered the king's service at the Escorial, where his intelligence and conduct seem to have made a favorable impression on those around him.

Philip chose him for a task that had been thoroughly neglected by the Conquistadors. The King probably sensed that the natural plant and animal resources of the region would eventually far outweigh the value of its gold and silver. Some 60,000 ducats were placed at the disposal of Hernandez and he was given the title of Protomedico, First Physician of the Indies. In 1570, together with his son, he sailed on an expedition meant to last five years. The time allotted seemed as ample as the funds, but both Philip and Hernandez had underestimated the prodigious quantities of material to be dealt with.

Luckily for Hernandez, the Aztecs had devised a system of naming plants which took into account their habitat and their properties, otherwise his work would have been impossibly difficult. As it was he was able to enlist guides, artists, herbalists, and physicians, all native, who acquainted him directly with the *materia medica* of the country. The Aztecs had developed extensive botanical gardens, zoos containing the animals, birds, and reptiles found in every corner of their realm, and had made collections of natural oddities and minerals, so that Hernandez was easily able to get a clear picture of Mexico's natural history. A further benefit was the fact that much of this had been set down in writing, and the pictographic symbols were still understood by the more educated natives.

The work of the expedition, however, was not confined to sedentary examination of codices, or to conducting interviews with those who knew the native plants, animals, and minerals. Much of it entailed travelling from place to place,

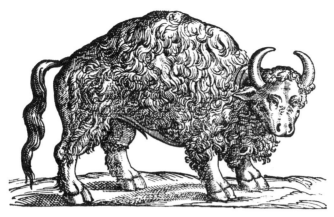

FIGURE 107. Taurus Mexicanus. The Taurus mexicanus of Hernandez is the familiar American bison, *Bos bison*, which once covered the plains in vast numbers from northern Canada to Mexico. The young animal's horns are sharply pointed and almost black, growing blunter and grayer with age. The animals are bare of their coats by the end of June, just in time to be plagued by flies and heat, but they have new, rich coats by December. (From Hernandez's *Rerum Medicarum* . . . Rome, V. Mascardi, 1651. Original size 5 ³/₄" wide × 4 ¹/₄" high.)

whether in steaming coastal jungles, chilly highlands, or parched desert areas. It was a physically exhausting task, with every risk of losing one's health. There were swarms of insects and poor sanitary conditions, and Hernandez emerged from the experience a debilitated man. On one occasion, he experimented on himself with *chupire*, one of the poisonous Euphorbiaceae, and almost died after swallowing some of its blistering latex. Its violent quality can be guessed at from one of its popular names, "planta del fuego," the plant of fire. The effect must have been very like a double cocktail of poison ivy.

Throughout his investigations Hernandez was careful to record the Mexican names of whatever plants he examined, whether in Tarascan, Michoacan, Aztec, or any other native tongue. Because of such records his *Rerum Medicarum Novae Hispaniae Thesaurus* (Treasury of the Medicinal Things of New Spain) is a valuable source of information about the ethnobotany of the region. In his pages are descriptions of

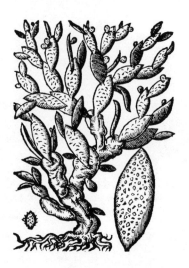

FIGURE 108. Opuntia. The cactus seen here is one of the Opuntias, a native of the New World, as are all cacti. This cactus quickly became naturalized through the entire Mediterranean region. One member of the genus, *O. ficus-indica*, produces the edible prickly pear which was widely cultivated in southern Europe. Opuntias are hardy. One kind, *O. humifusa*, has even extended its range as far north as Massachusetts. (From Hernandez's *Rerum Medicarum* . . . Rome, V. Mascardi, 1651. Original size 2 ³/₄" wide × 4" high.)

the dahlia, which the Aztecs had brought to a high point of development, and of the tigridia, in which many European herbalists refused to believe (although they could readily swallow tales about the goose-tree or the vegetable-lamb). There is also a description of ololiuhqui, a hallucinogen used by the priests when they wished to communicate with their gods or to receive visions. A chapter on Jasper, or "bloodstone," shows it was used in a powdered form for exactly the same purpose that Europeans used it for, stopping hemorrhages. But copal, which the Indians burned as incense, was used in Europe as a protective varnish. There were descriptions of bison, 'possums, and even of a one-horned dragon, the chapter on which was dedicated to Cardinal Barberini. The dragon was of course a mixture of bird, beast, and reptile put together by some ingenious native. It was outfitted with a pair of scaly wings perhaps to compensate it for possessing only a pair of weak forelegs to get about upon.

One product Hernandez made certain to include was Guaiacum, sometimes called Holy Wood, which was then believed to be an absolute cure for the pox (syphilis), a disease that every European country claimed had originated in a neighboring land. When the bark was discovered not to be an antisyphilitic as supposed, but simply a stimulant and diaphoretic, interest in it waned as rapidly as it had risen. Another item Hernandez expatiated upon was the paper used by the Aztecs in compiling the great codices that held their histories, legends, and statistics. The paper was actually the bark from different species of fig trees, some white and highly polished, some yellowish in hue. Reams of it poured into the capitol city annually from every part of Mexico. Cuernavaca alone provided as many as 160,000 sheets per year. Unluckily only 17 pre-Columbian codices, 3 Mayan and 14 Aztec, have survived from out of the mountainous pile of records and books that were in existence at the time of the Conquest.

Having gathered all of his material, Hernandez, at great sacrifice to himself and his purse once the official funds ran out, remained in Mexico another two years to revise his work and complete his mission. During that time he had three or four copies made from his manuscript, and purposely left them behind when he returned to Spain in 1577. Not a single copy survived.

Nor was the ultimate fate of the manuscript he presented to Philip II any better. The copious text had been gathered into 16 folio-sized volumes, 6 of text and 10 of drawings. In addition, they contained 19 other manuscripts by Hernandez, including a Spanish translation of the 37 books of Pliny. Gratefully received by Philip, who had earlier offered Hernandez the leadership of an expedition to Peru in gratitude for his herculean efforts, the manuscript was honored with sumptuous bindings of gold-tooled leather, fitted with clasps, corners, and ornaments of solid silver, and then buried in the library of the Escorial. Since Hernandez had refused the Peruvian expedition on the grounds not only of ill health but of his desire to be in Spain to see his masterwork through the press, this unexpected treatment was something of a blow. The worst, however, was still to come, for his book languished there unpublished until years after his death in 1587 at about the age of 73.

Philip finally did resolve to publish some of the more useful portions of the manuscript, and authorized another of his physicians, Dr. Nardo Antonio Recchi of Montecorvo, a small town near Naples, to make an extract. That too remained unpublished during Recchi's lifetime, but following his death, the manuscript he had carved out of the Hernandez text passed to his nephew, a lawyer named Petililo, who also lived in Montecorvo. Later another extract was made from the original by the Jesuit, Juan Eusebio Nieremberg, for his 1635 publication titled *Historia naturae maxime peregrinae*. Manuscript copies of the Recchi condensation continued to be made, and the botanical portion of one of these was found and published at Madrid in 1790. The original Hernandez manuscript in the Escorial, including all of the drawings, perished in the fire that devastated the palace in 1671. Only a few fragments survived the flames.

FIGURE 109. Title page of *Rerum Medicarum*. The title page of the *Rerum Medicarum Novae Hispaniae Thesaurus* (The Treasury of the Medicinal Things of New Spain) seems to have needed a great deal of space to give credit to everyone involved in its production. None of Hernandez's actual text appears, only the summaries made by Recchio and the added remarks of Terrentio, Fabri, and Colonna. The indices make use of the native names, and pose difficulties for readers unfamiliar with the various Indian tongues of Mexico. (From Hernandez's *Rerum Medicarum . . .* Rome, V. Mascardi, 1651. Reduced from original size, 8" wide × 11 3/4" high.)

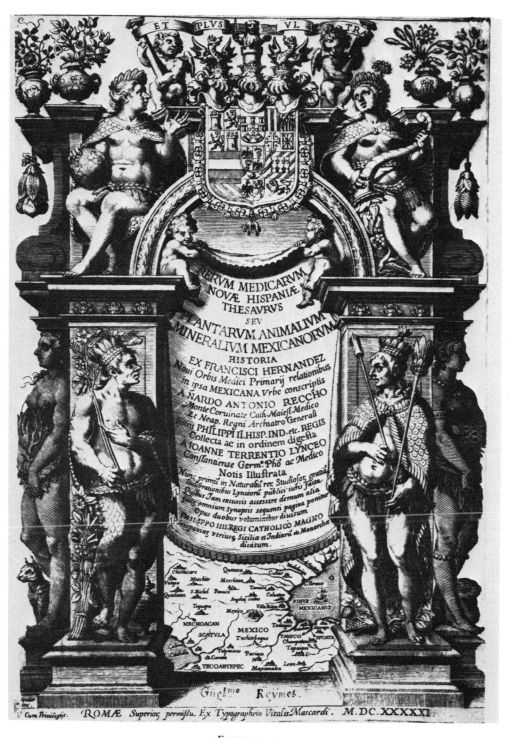

ET PLVS VLTR.

RERVM MEDICARVM
NOVÆ HISPANIÆ
THESAVRVS
SEV
PLANTARVM ANIMALIVM
MINERALIVM MEXICANORVM
HISTORIA
EX FRANCISCI HERNANDEZ
Noui Orbis Medici Primarij relationibus
in ipsa MEXICANA Vrbe conscriptis
A NARDO ANTONIO RECCHO
Monte Coruinate Cath. Maiest. Medico
Et Neap. Regni Archiatro Generali
iussu PHILIPPI II. HISP. IND. etc. REGIS
Collecta ac in ordinem digesta
A IOANNE TERRENTIO LYNCEO
Constantiense Germ° Phő ac Medico
Notis Illustrata
Nunc primū in Naturalū rer. Studiosoꝝ gratiā
lucubrationibus Lynceorū publici iuris facta.
Quibus Iam excussis accessere demum alia
quoꝛ omnium Synopsis sequenti pagina ponitur
Opus duobus voluminibus diuisum
PHILIPPO IIII. REGI CATHOLICO MAGNO
Hispaniaꝛ Vtriusꝗ Siciliæ et Indiarū & Monarchæ
dicatum.

Gumeca. Mꝛ
Chichicare Culiaca. Mꝛ
Volga Merchiar Meschtan. C. Bianco
Quazatlan S. Michel Panuco Tonatla. Mꝛ Cꝛlaqua
Tapaga Axoples cixtin VillaRica. Mꝛ SINVS
Mexico MEXICANVS
MECHOACAN Tedaca
SCATVLA MEXICO Tabasco
Tuslatlabeque Champaton IVCATA
Tecpan Tequanes Paciaco Tiquian Mꝛ
C. Canela Sella Leon Arboꝛ
TECOANTEPEC Maxamala.

Gulielmo Reymes.

Cum Priuilegijs. ROMÆ Superioꝝ permissu. Ex Typographeio Vitalis Mascardi. M.DC.XXXXXI.

FIGURE 109.

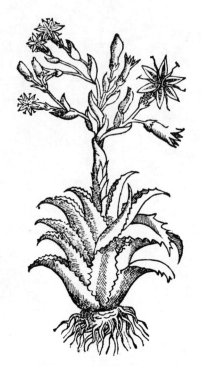

FIGURE 110. Metl. The Metl of Hernandez was one of the Agaves, New World plants that superficially resembled the Old World Aloes but had no botanical or chemical relationship to them. Called the Maguey in Mexico, this plant provides soap and fibers for a strong thread that may be woven into a coarse, useful cloth. When its juices are fermented they become an intoxicating beverage known as pulque. (From Hernandez's *Rerum Medicarum* . . . Rome, V. Mascardi, 1651. Original size 2 ⁵/₁₆" wide × 4 ¹/₂" high.)

In the meantime, one Fray Francisco Ximenez, who had been an apothecary in Florida but had later emigrated to Mexico and entered a religious order, came into possession of a copy of Recchi's manuscript. Recognizing its value, he translated it from Latin into Spanish and published it in Mexico for the first time anywhere in 1615. Meanwhile in Italy the nephew of Recchi, who had inherited his uncle's manuscript, sold it to the Accademia Lincei, a scientific society founded at Naples by Prince Federigo Cesi. The group began preparing it for the press and even managed to have a few copies printed in 1628, but due to a lack of funds the printing was halted. The situation had not changed by the time of Prince Cesi's death two years later in 1630, so the project remained shelved until 1651. In that year a successful attempt was made to enlist financial aid from the Spanish government, and a two-volume edition, bearing many woodcuts prepared from copies of the Aztec artists' drawings, finally appeared.

A change of country, new editors, new sponsorship, and 74 years was all it took to get Hernandez's work published, but of course at the sacrifice of his original text. It was a belated and inadequate tribute to the first natural history of Mexico, and the record of the first official scientific expedition to the New World, but we must be grateful for the remnant we possess. As one bibliographer said of Hernandez's writings, they seemed to have a curse upon them. Along with Job, Hernandez might well have said, "My desire is, that the Almighty would answer me, and that mine adversary had written a book."

BIBLIOGRAPHIC NOTES

1st edition: 1615, edited by Fray Francisco Ximenez, printed by Diego Lopez Davalos in Mexico, no town given.

2nd edition: 1628, edited by Nardo Antonio Recchi, Ioanne Terrentio, Ioanne Fabro, and Fabio Columna, printed at Rome by J. Mascardi. Very rare.

3rd edition: 1651, same editors, at Rome by V. Mascardi. This is the only complete version with all the illustrations.

4th edition: 1790, edited by Casimir Gomez Ortega, and printed by Ibarrae Heredum at Madrid. Has complete text of botanical portions only. No illustrations.

5th edition: 1888, edited by Dr. Nicolas Leon, printed by La Escuela de Artes for Jose R. Bravo at Morelia, Mexico. This is a reprint of the 1615 Ximenez edition.

6th edition: 1942 at Mexico City by the Instituto de Biologia de la Universidad Nacional Autonoma de Mexico at the University Press. This is an annotated reprint of the Ximenez edition, with illustrations added from the 1651 edition.

Glossary

ALEMBIC:	An apparatus used in distillation. It consisted of a cucurbit (a gourd-shaped vessel) that held the material to be distilled, and a head that capped the cucurbit. Vapors were condensed in the head and conveyed by a tube to a separate container called the receiver.
AROMATICS:	Plant- or animal-based materials of medicine with agreeable odors. The scents were thought to have healing or disease-preventing properties.
BOLE:	Earth or clay, often astringent in nature, which was supplied to physicians and apothecaries in a tablet form that bore a seal identifying its place of origin.
BRUISE:	To pound herbs lightly.
CODEX:	A group of codices bound together.
CODICE:	A volume made of separate pages, rather than a scroll.
DEGREE:	A noticeable difference in the strength and effect of a medicinal substance. Rated in terms of hot or cold, moist or dry, the degrees ranged from temperate (perfectly neutral), to mild (or first degree), to the strongest possible (or fourth degree). Items in the fourth degree were usually poisonous or caustic.

DOCTRINE OF SIGNATURES:	The theory stating that each plant bore a visible mark that revealed its intended use. Plants with sharply cut leaves or thorns would cure bites, while others with heart-shaped leaves, bulbs, or fruits would be useful in cardiac disorders, etc.
FEMININE HERBS:	Those herbs with weaker characteristics than other plants related to or resembling them.
GHOST:	In bibliography, an edition that has been entered into the record but that never existed.
HERBAL:	A book concerned with the materials of medicine, especially of a botanical origin, although animal and mineral substances may also be included.
HERBALIST:	One skilled in the finding, identification, preparation, and use of medicinal herbs.
HUMOUR:	One of the four fluids produced by and within the body from its nutrients. They were thought to correspond to the four elements of air, water, fire, and earth, and were called blood (hot and moist), phlegm (cold and moist), choler (hot and dry), and melancholia (cold and dry). If they remained in balance the body was healthy, but if an imbalance developed, ill health followed.
INCUNABULA:	Books printed in the cradle days of printing, c. 1454–1500. From "cunabula," the Latin for cradle.
MAGISTER:	Title given to a Master who taught any branch of learning.
MASCULINE HERBS:	Herbs with stronger color, taste, and smell, or with more vigorous growth than other similar ones, which were known as "feminine herbs."
MATULA:	A glass vessel bearing a series of marks. It was used for diagnostic examination of urine, the marks indicating favorable or unfavorable levels for sediments, floating particles, or clouds that could be seen in the urine.

MEDICINAL WATERS: Fluids extracted by distillation from herbs or other medicinal substances.

MELANCHOLIA: A Greek word for black choler, one of the four humours of the body, which was thought to originate in the spleen and to be the cause of insanity.

MELANCHOLY: *See* Melancholia.

PALIMPSEST: From the Greek words for "scraped again," referring to the practice of reusing parchment by scraping away the text that had been originally written upon it. The legible traces so left have often preserved complete texts that would otherwise have been lost.

PARCHMENT: Sheepskin prepared for writing purposes by scraping the wool and fleshy remnants from a stretched hide. Name derives from Pergamon, an early center for supply of the product.

PELICAN: A vessel with a downward curving spout, often used in distillation.

PHARMACOPEIA: A book of drug substances and medicinal preparations, usually but not always issued by official authority and providing recognized standards.

PHLEBOTOMY: Venesection, the practice of opening veins to draw off blood. Often used in early medicine in conjunction with or as a prelude to purging, to rid the body of evil humours.

PHYSIC: The practice of medicine; not merely a purgative, as the term indicates today. Physic referred to nonsurgical treatment of disease.

PLASTER: A pastelike concoction smeared onto the affected area.

PLATE: An etched or engraved piece of metal bearing a design that is to be printed. The term is also used for the prints struck from the metal plate.

PRIVILEGE: An early form of legal protection for publications, similar to the present-day copyright. It was issued to authors and publishers for a definite period of time either by royal authority or by some other governing body.

RETORT: A distiller's vessel similar to the pelican, but with a tapering neck bent at a right angle to its flasklike body.

SEALED EARTH: Special clays or earths bearing the recognized seal or official device of the town or region in which they were either found or prepared; *see* Bole.

SHARP HERBS: Plants with a very pungent odor or flavor, such as mustard.

SIMPLE: A single, unmixed, uncompounded medicinal substance; usually a plant, though minerals and animal products could also be so named.

SIGNATURE: *See* Doctrine of Signatures.

STAMP: To pound herbs into a paste in a mortar.

STILL-ROOM: A room in a manor house wherein herbs were distilled to provide medicinal fluids. The room was also used to dry, prepare, and store herbs for future use. Some were used in cookery.

UROSCOPY: Diagnosis by means of visual examination of the color, clarity, and other visible characteristics of urine. Its claims became increasingly exaggerated before it was abandoned as a false system.

VELLUM: Calfskin scraped, stretched, and prepared for writing purposes. Lamb and kid were also used. From the old French word "veel," for calf, originally from the Latin "vitellus," a little calf.

VIRTUES: The specific medicinal properties of herbs or other medicaments. For example, "It hath a healing virtue for green [fresh] wounds," or "It hath the virtue of breaking the stone [shattering or powdering kidney and bladder stones]."

WOODBLOCK: *See* Woodcut.

WOODCUT: A block of wood cut so as to form a raised surface that will print a design when inked and placed in a press. It is also the name for prints so produced. It was the earliest means of illustrating printed books.

WORT: Any medicinal plant; derived from the Anglo-Saxon "wyrt," meaning herb or root.

Bibliography

Albertus Magnus (Meyer, E., and Jessen, C., eds.): *Historia naturalis*. Pars XVIII, De Vegetabilibus, Libri VII. Berolini, 1867.

[Pseudo-] Albertus Magnus: *De secretis mulierum libellus*. Strassburg, 1607.

—— *De secretis naturae, liber aggregationis*. Venice, not before 1487.

—— *Naturalia*. Strassburg, 1548.

Antonius Musa: *De Herba Vetonica Liber Uno*. Tiguria, 1537.

Apulei: *De Medicaminibus Herbarum Liber Uno*. Tiguria, 1537.

Arber, Agnes: *Herbals, Their Origin and Evolution*. Cambridge, 1938.

Aston, Margaret E.: "The Fiery Trigon Conjunction." *Isis*, Vol. 61, pt. 2, No. 207 (1970).

Avery, A. G., Satina, S. and Rietsema, J.: *Blakeslee: The Genus "Datura."* New York, 1959.

Banckes, Rycharde: *An Herbal*. Facsimile of the 1525 London ed., edited by Larkey and Pyles. New York, 1941.

Bartholomaeus Anglicus: *De proprietatibus rerum*. Lyons, 1483.

Bauhin, C.: *Pinax Theatri Botanici*. Basileae, 1623.

Bayon, H. P.: *Masters of Salerno (in Science, Medicine, and History)*. London and New York, 1953.

Beardsley, Katherine: "Hallucinogens: Some Notes on Their Origins, Uses, and Social Implications." *The Herbarist*, No. 36 (1970).

Beck, Claus: *Studien über Gestalt und Ursprung des Circa instans.* . . . Wurzburg, 1940.

Blancardi (Blankaart), Stephen: *Lexicon Novum Medicarum.* Lugduni Batavorum, 1701.

Blunt, Wilfrid: *The Art of Botanical Illustration.* London, 1950.

Bock, Hieronymous: *Kreüter Buch.* Strassburg, 1539.

Brock, Arthur J. (M.D.): *Greek Medicine.* Trans. of Greek writings. New York, 1929.

Brodin, Gösta, ed.: *Agnus Castus, a Middle English Herbal. . . .* Uppsala and Cambridge, Mass., 1950.

Brooklyn Botanic Garden: *Handbook on Herbs.* Baltimore, 1958.

Brunfels, O.: *Herbarum Vivae Eicones.* Strassburg, 1530.

Brunschwig, Hieronymous: *Das Buch zu Distillieren.* Strassburg, 1519.

Brunschweig, Jerome (Andrewe trans.): *The Vertuose Boke of Dystyllacyon of the Waters of All Maner of Herbes.* London, 1527.

Budge, Sir Ernest Wallis: *The Divine Origin of the Craft of The Herbalist.* London, 1928.

—— *Syrian Anatomy, Pathology and Therapeutics, or "The Book of Medicines."* 2 vols. London and New York, 1913.

Burgess, E. S.: *Memoirs of The Torrey Botanical Club.* Vol. X: *History of Pre-Clusian Botany in its Relation to Aster.* New York, 1902.

Camus, Giulio: *L'Opera Salernitana "Circa instans" ed Il Testo Primitivo del Grant Herbier en Francoys.* Modena, 1886.

Castiglioni, Arturo (Krumbhaar trans.): *The History of Medicine.* New York, 1947.

Clendening, Logan (M.D.): *Source Book of Medical History.* New York, 1942.

Coats, Alice M.: *Flowers and Their Histories.* London, 1956.

Cockayne, O.: *Leechdoms, Wortcunning and Starcraft of Early England.* London, 1864.

Coles, William: *Adam in Eden.* London, 1657.

Colonna, Fabio: *Phytobasanos.* Naples, 1592.

Conrad von Megenberg: *Buch der Natur.* Augsburg, 1475.

Coon, Nelson: "The Fragrant Herb Garden." *The Herbarist,* No. 32 (1966).

Crescenzi, Pietro de (Sansovino trans.): *Le Cose Della Villa.* Venice, 1564.

Crescenzi, Pietro de (Lo'nferigno trans.): *Trattato della Agricoltura.* Bologna, 1784.

Crisp, Sir Frank (Paterson ed.): *Medieval Gardens.* London, 1924.

Cronquist, Arthur: *Introductory Botany.* New York, 1961.

Culpeper, N.: *Culpeper's Complete Herbal.* Reprint of 1733 ed. London, 1955.
—— *A Physical Directory.* 3rd ed. London, 1651.
Da Orta, Garcia (Markham trans.): *Colloquies on the Simples and Drugs of India.* London, 1913.
De Ropp, Robert S.: *Drugs and the Mind.* New York, 1957.
Dictionary of National Biography (ed. by Stephen and Lee). London and New York, 1908.
Dioscorides (Gunther-Goodyer trans.): *De Materia Medica.* Oxford, 1934.
—— *Materia medica.* Juliana Anicia Codex, Codex Vindobonensis Med. Gr. 1, facsimile. Graz, Austria, 1970.
Dodoens, Rembert (Lyte trans.): *The Nievve Herball.* London, 1578.
Durante, C.: *Herbario Nuovo.* Venice, 1717.
Earle, John: *English Plant Names from the Xth to the XVth Century.* Oxford, 1880.
Eger, Fay B.: Letter to *The Herbarist. The Herbarist,* No. 33 (1967).
Emmart, Emily Walcott: *The Badianus Manuscript.* Codex Barberini, Latin 241, Vatican Library. (An Aztec Herbal of 1552). Baltimore, 1940.
Encyclopaedia Britannica, 11th ed. New York, 1910.
Fernie, W. T., (M.D.): *Herbal Simples.* 2nd ed. Philadelphia, 1897.
Fischer, Hermann: *Mittelalterliche Pflanzenkunde.* München, 1929.
Folkard, Richard, Jr.: *Plant Lore, Legends and Lyrics.* London, 1884.
Freeman, Margaret B.: *Herbs for the Medieval Household.* New York, 1943.
Fuchs, Leonhart: *Commentaries tres excellens de l'hystoire des plantes.* Paris, 1549.
—— *De Historia Stirpium.* Basle, 1542.
Garrison, Fielding H., and Morton, L. T.: *A Medical Bibliography.* London, 1943.
Gates, William, ed.: *De la Cruz-Badiano Aztec Herbal.* Baltimore, 1939.
Gerard, John: *The Herball.* London, 1597.
Giacosa, Piero: *Magistri Salernitani Nondum Editi.* Torino, 1901.
Goff, F. R.: *Incunabula in American Libraries,* 3rd census . . . New York, 1964.
Greene, Edward Lee: *Landmarks of Botanical History.* Washington, D.C., 1909.
Grieve, M. and Leyel, C. F.: *A Modern Herbal.* 2 vols. London and New York, 1931.

Gunther, Robert T., ed.: *The Herbal of Apuleius, from the Early XII Century Ms. formerly in the Abbey of Bury St. Edmunds. Ms. Bodley 130.* Oxford, 1925.

Hatton, Richard G.: *Handbook of Plant and Floral Ornament.* New York, 1960.

Hawks, Ellison: *Pioneers of Plant Study.* Freeport, N.Y., 1969.

Henschel, A. W. E. Th.: *Des Cod. Salernitanus der Stadtbibliothek zu Breslau.* Janus, Vol. 1. Reprint of orig. 1846 ed. Leipzig, 1931.

Henslow, G.: *Medical Works of the XIVth Century.* London, 1899.

Henslow, G. (Rev. Prof.): *The Plants of the Bible.* London, 1906.

Herbarius latinus. Vicenza, 1491.

Hernandez, F.: *Cuatro Libros de la Naturaleza.* Morelia, 1888.

—— *Rerum Medicarum Novae Hispaniae.* Rome, 1651.

Hildegarde of Bingen: *Opera omnia.* Paris, 1882.

—— *Physica.* Argentorati, 1533.

Hind, Arthur M.: *An Introduction to a History of Woodcut.* 2 vols. New York, 1963.

Histoire des drogues espisceries, et decertains medicamens simples, qui naissent és Indies et en Amerique. Lyon, 1619.

Hoffer, A., and Osmond, H.: *The Hallucinogens.* New York and London, 1967.

Hortus Sanitatis. Strassburg, 1497.

Hudson, Noel: *An Early English Version of the Hortus Sanitatis, a facsimile of The Noble Lyfe and Natures of Man . . .* Ed. of Antwerp, 1510. London, 1954.

Hunger, F. W. T.: *The Herbal of Pseudo-Apuleius, from the IX Century Ms. in the Abbey of Monte Cassino [Codex Casinensis 97] together with the first printed edition of Joh. Phil. de Lignamine [Ed. Prin. Rome 1481], both in facsimile.* Leyden, 1935.

Hunt Botanical Catalogue, The. 2 vols. (Jane Quinby, comp.) Pittsburgh, Pa., 1958.

Hunter, Dard: *Papermaking: The History and Technique of an Ancient Craft.* New York, 1943.

Isidore of Seville: *Etymologiarum.* Oxford, 1971.

Ivins, William M., Jr.: *How Prints Look.* Boston, 1958.

Karnick, C. R.: "True Identity of Soma Plant. . . ." *Quarterly Journal of Crude Drug Research.* Vol. IX, No. 4 (1969).

Klebs, Arnold C., M.D.: *A Catalogue of Early Herbals. . . .* Lugano, Switzerland, 1925.

—— *Incunabula Lists.* (Papers of the Bibliographical Society of America Vol. XII.) Chicago, 1918.

—— *Incunabula Scientifica et Medica.* Vol. IV. Osiris, 1937.

Kramer, Samuel Noah: *From the Tablets of Sumer.* Indian Hills, Colorado, 1956.

Kreig, Margaret B.: *Green Medicine.* Chicago, New York, San Francisco, 1964.

Kristeller, P. O.: "The School of Salerno." *Bulletin of the History of Medicine.* Vol. 17. 1945.

Krutch, Joseph Wood: *Herbal.* New York, 1965.

La Wall, Charles H.: *Four Thousand Years of Pharmacy.* Philadelphia and London, 1927.

Lawrence, George H. M.: "Herbals, the End of an Era." *The Herbarist,* No. 35 (1969).

Leach, M. and Friedman, J., eds.: *Standard Dictionary of Folklore, Mythology and Legend.* New York, 1949.

Leclerc, Lucien: *Histoire de la Médecine Arabe.* New York, 1971.

Le Grant Herbier. Paris. Not before 1521.

Leighton, Ann: *Early American Gardens.* Boston, 1970.

Levey, Martin: *Early Arabic Pharmacology.* Leiden, 1973.

Lewin, Louis: *Phantastica, Narcotic and Stimulating Drugs.* New York, 1931.

Leyel, Mrs. C. F.: *The Magic of Herbs.* New York, 1926.

Linné, Carl von (Hort trans.): *Critica Botanica.* London, 1938.

—— *Materia Medica.* (Schreber ed.) Lipsiae et Erlangae, 1772.

Lonitzer, Adam: *Kreütterbuch.* Frankfurt am Main, 1557.

Lowndes, William Thomas: *Bibliographer's Manual of English Literature.* Revised and enlarged by Henry G. Bohn. 6 vols. London, 1890.

Lyons, A. B. (M.D.): *Plant Names Scientific and Popular.* Detroit, 1900.

McDaniel, W. B. 2nd: "Early Illustrated Herbals in the Library of the College of Physicians of Philadelphia." *The Herbarist,* No. 28 (1962).

MacKinney, L. C.: " 'Dynamidia' in Medieval Medical Literature." *Isis,* Vol. 24, pt. 2, No. 68 (Feb. 1936).

Macer Floridus: *De virtutibus herbarum.* Venice, 1506.

Maplet, John: *A Greene Forest.* (Reprint of 1567 ed.) London, 1930.

Matthews, Leslie G.: *History of Pharmacy in Britain.* Edinburgh and London, 1962.

Mattioli, Pier Andrea: *Commentarii.* Venice, 1564.

Medicina Antiqua Libri Quattuor Medicinae Codex Vindobonensis 93. (With commentary by C. Talbot and F. Unterkircher) Graz, Austria, 1972.

Mesue: *Opera quae extant omnia*. Venice, 1562.

Meyer, Ernst: *Geschichte der Botanik*. 4 vols. Koenigsberg, 1857.

Meyerhof, Max: "Thirty-three clinical observations by Rhazes (ca. 900 A.D.)." *Isis*, Vol. 23, pt. 2, No. 66 (1935).

Moldenke, H. N. and A. L.: *Plants of the Bible*. Waltham, Mass., 1952.

Monardes, N. (Frampton trans.): *Joyfull Newes Out of the Newe Found Worlde*. London and New York, 1925.

Mowat, J. L. G., ed.: *Alphita: A Medico-Botanical Glossary*. Oxford, 1887.

—— *Synonyma Bartholomei*. Oxford, 1882.

Moyses, Rabbi (Moses ben Maimon Maimonides): *Tractatus de Regimen Sanitatis ad Soldanum Regem*. Augsburg, 1518.

Munting, Abraham: *Waare Oeffening der Planten*. Amsterdam, 1682.

Nadkarni, K. M.: *Indian Materia Medica*. 3rd ed. 2 vols. Bombay, 1955.

Nissen, Claus: *Die Botanische Buchillustration ihre Geschichte und Bibliographie*. Stuttgart, 1951.

Nissen, Claus: *Herbals of Five Centuries*. Zurich, Munich, Olten, 1958.

Nordenskiöld, Erik (Bucknall-Eyre trans.): *The History of Biology, a Survey*. New York, London, 1928.

Parkinson, John: *Paradisi in Sole Paradisus Terrestris*. London, 1629.

—— *Theatrum Botanicum*. London, 1640.

Peck, Harry Thurston, ed.: *Harper's Dictionary of Classical Antiquities and Literature*. Reprint ed. New York, 1963.

Platearius, Matthaeus: *Circa instans* (in Serapion). Venice, 1497.

—— *Expositionibus et glossis super Antidotarium parvum Nicolai* (in Mesue). Venice, 1562.

Pliny (Loeb Classical Library ed.): *Historia naturalis*. 10 vols. Cambridge, Mass., 1938.

Pliny (Bostock and Riley trans.): *Natural History*. 6 vols. London, 1855–57.

Pomet, Pierre: *A Compleat History of Druggs*. London, 1737.

Porta, Gianbattista: *Natural Magick*. Facsimile of 1st English ed. New York, 1957.

Pritzel, G. A.: *Thesaurus Literaturae Botanicae*. Milano, 1950.

Quincy, John: *Pharmacopeia Officinalis*. London, 1720.

Raven, Charles E.: *John Ray, Naturalist, His Life & Works*. Cambridge, 1950.

Reed, Howard S.: *Short History of the Plant Sciences.* Waltham, Mass., 1942.

Rees, Abraham: *The Cyclopedia.* Philadelphia and New York, 1810–1824.

Rohde, E. S.: *The Old English Herbals.* New York, 1922.

—— *Shakespeare's Wild Flowers.* . . . London, 1935.

Saint-Lager, Dr.: "Recherches sur les Anciens Herbaria." *Annales de la Societe Botanique de Lyon,* Vol. XII (Lyon, 1885).

Sarton, George: *The History of Science.* 2 vols. New York, 1970.

—— *Introduction to the History of Science.* 3 vols. Baltimore, 1927–1948.

—— "Scientific Incunabula." *Osiris,* Vol. V. (Bruges, 1938).

Schenk, Gustav: *The Book of Poisons.* New York, 1955.

Schmid, A.: *Ueber alte Kraüterbücher.* Bern and Leipzig, 1939.

Schröder, Johann: *Pharmacopëia medico-chymica.* Lugduni, 1649.

Scribonius Largus: *Compositiones Medicae.* Patavii, 1655.

Serapion, Jr.: *Breviarum medicinae.* Venice, 1497.

—— *Liber Serapionis agregatus in medicinis simplicibus.* Milan, 1473.

Shewell-Cooper, W. E.: *Plants and Fruits of the Bible.* London, 1962.

Shlomoh, Rabbi Gershon ben (Bodenheimer trans.): *The Gate of Heaven (Shaár ha-Shamayim).* Jerusalem, 1953.

Singer, Charles: *From Magic to Science.* New York, 1928.

—— "Herbals in Antiquity." *Journal of Hellenic Studies,* Vol. XLVII (London, n.d.).

—— *A Short History of Biology.* Oxford, 1931.

Skinner, C. M.: *Myths and Legends of Flowers, Trees, Fruits and Plants in All Ages and in All Climes.* Philadelphia 1925.

Smith, Frederick Porter: *Contributions Towards the Materia Medica and Natural History of China.* Shanghai and London, 1871.

Sprague, T. A., and Nelmes, E.: "The Herbal of Leonhart Fuchs." *Linnean Society Journal,* Vol. XLVIII (London, 1931).

Sprague, T. A.: "The Herbal of Otto Brunfels." *Linnean Society Journal* (Botany), Vol. XLVIII (1928).

Starkenstein, W.: "Ein Beitrag zur 'Circa instans'–Frage." *Sudhoff's Archiv,* Vol. 27 (1935).

Stillwell, M. B.: *Incunabula and Americana 1450–1800.* New York, 1961.

Strabo, Walahfrid: *Hortulus.* Pittsburgh, 1966.

Strong, Caroline B.: "The Strewing Herbs." *The Herbarist,* No. 29 (1963).

Sudhoff, K.: "Die Salernitaner Handschrift in Breslau." *Archiv fur Geschichter der Medizin,* Vol. 12 (1920).

Theophrastus, (Hort trans.): *Enquiry into Plants.* 2 vols. London, 1916.

Thistleton-Dyer, T. F.: *The Folklore of Plants.* London, 1889.

Thompson, C. J. S.: *The Mystery and the Art of the Apothecary.* London, 1929.

Thompson, R. C.: *A Dictionary of Assyrian Botany.* London, 1949.

Thorndike, Lynn, ed.: *The Herbal of Rufinus.* Chicago, 1945.

Thurneisser, Leonhard: *Historia sive Descriptio Plantarum Omnium.* Berlin, 1578.

Trimen, Henry, and Thistleton-Dyer, Wm. T.: *Flora of Middlesex.* London, 1869.

Turner, William: *A New Herball.* Collen, 1568.

U.S. National Library of Medicine: *Catalogue of XVIth Century Printed Books in the U.S. National Library of Medicine.* Washington, D.C., 1967.

von Haller, Albert: *Bibliotheca Botanica.* 2 vols. Tiguri, 1771.

Woelfel, H.: "Das Arzneidrogenbuch 'Circa instans,' in einer Fassung des 13 Jahrhunderts aus der Universitäts-bibliothek Erlangen." Dissertation, Friedr. Wilhelm Univ., Berlin, 1939.

Index

Abraham ben' Shemtob, 40
Abraham Tortuosensis, *see* Abraham ben' Shemtob
Accademia dei Lincei, 194, 216, 243
Achates, Leonardus, 88
Achilles, 24
Aconitum napellus, 171
Aemilius Macer, 30
Amatus Lusitanos, 168
Anazarba, 8
Andrewe, Laurens, 117
Anguillara, Luigi, 168
Anicius Olybrius, 11
Anise, 109, 111
Antidotarium of Nicholas of Salerno, 48
Antwerp, 177, 180, 206, 209
Apuleius, 23-26, 29
Arabic translated in Spain, 42
Arber, Agnes, 32
Arbolayre, 98-99
Areius, 8
Aristotle, 64, 196
Arnaldus de Villanova, 84

Arndes, Steffan, 97
Arnold de Bruxella, 35
Arnoullet, Balthasar, 147
Arum, 76
Ashmolean Library, 65
Astrology, 181-86, 196, 199
Augsburg, 72, 81, 96-97, 114, 162
Avicenna, 44, 84, 104

Bämler, Hans, 81
Banckes' *Herbal,* 148
Barbarus, Hermolaus, 22
Barnacle Goose, 161, 217
Bartholomä, Daniel, 162
Bartholomaeus Anglicus, 57, 59-65
Bascarini, Nicolo de, 164, 171
Basel, 60, 65, 97, 128, 145-46, 172, 177, 181-82
Beck, Renatus, 112
Beham, Hans, 157
Benalius, Bernardinus, 112
Berlin, 182, 186

Berne, 124, 129
Berthelin, I., 200
Besançon, 98, 105
Bevilacqua, Simon, 88
Bezoar Stone, 161-62, 208
Birckman, Arnold, 152, 155
Blunt, Wilfrid, 32
Bock, Hieronymus (Jerome), 130-36; biography, 132; botanical education, 132; botanical innovations, 130-34; dislike of his name, 134; experiment with ferns, 136
Böckelheim, 51
Bologna, 69, 70
Bonetum, Locatellum, 50
Bonfadino, Bartholomeo, 192
Bonhomme, Jean, 88
Book trade, in 15th century, 92
Bostock and Riley, 22
Boswellia carteri, 30
Bouncing Bet, *see Saponaria officinalis*
Breslau Codex, 50
Briganti, Annibal, 209
Brunfels, Otto, 51, 121-29; biography of, 128-29; botanical inadequacies, 125-28; encourages Bock, 128
Brunschwig, Jerome (Hieronymus), 112, 113-19; the *Cirurgia*, 114-17; the *Distilierbuch*, 117; in Lonitzer's *Kreütterbuch*, 156; problems of his text, 113-14
Buch der Natur, 73-81; herbal section, 77; manuscripts of, 79; quotes from, 74-77; sources of, 74
Buch zu Distillieren, confusion about title, 113-14
Burgess, Edward Sanford, 49

Busbecq, Ogier, 10
Byzantium, 8-11

Cambridge University, 148-49
Camphor, 204
Camus, Giulio, 101-5
Cannabis sativa, 57
Cantimpré, Thomas de, 73-74
Carlinum, J. J., 217
Carrichter, Bartholomaeus, 185
Carthage, 24
Castigationes Plinianae, 22
Castor bean, 159
Caxton, William, 60
Charles II of Anjou, 70
Chiron, 24
Choulant, Ludwig, 34, 56
Circa instans, 45-50; authorship, 46, 48; contributions of, 49; earliest manuscripts, 49-50, 103; innovations, 45; purpose of, 45-46; relation to Le Grant Herbier, 98-99; source for Bartholomaeus Anglicus, 64; source for Crescenzi, 68-69; source for von Megenberg, 74; theories of Camus, 101-5; varying length, 48
Clemens Patavinus, 44
Clerical Medicine and Science, 52, 56, 73
Clusius, Carolus, 173-74, 209; collaborations, 175, 177; translations, 178, 206, 209
Cockayne, Oswald, 29
Codex Vindobonensis Med. Gr. I, 10, 15
Colin, Antoine, 209
Colle, 15
Collen, *see* Cologne
Cologne, 152, 155, 174, 182, 186

Colonna, Fabio, 194, 210-17, 243; botanical contributions, 216; death of, 217; edits Hernandez, 216; ends Barnacle Goose myth, 217; epilepsy cure, 211; etching, 213; invents musical instrument, 216; organizes Lincei, 216; use of register, 214-15; varied talents, 211

Coloquios, Los, 202-6, 209; breadth of, 205; cited in 19th century, 202; Goa editions, 206; list of editions, 209; translations of, 206

Coltsfoot, *see Tussilago farfara*

Commentarii of Mattioli, 166-68, 171-72; errors of, 168; expansion of Dioscorides, 169-71; illustrators of, 167; translations of, 171

Como, 20

Conrad von Megenberg, 73-81; biography, 73-74; observations of nature, 77; paralysis of, 81

Constantine, 8

Constantinople, 14

Coriander, *see Coriandrum sativum*

Coriandrum sativum, 87

Corn, *see Zea mays*

Cotes, Thomas, 234

Cotier, Gabriel, 172

Cousteau, Jacques, 26

Cranchsnabel, *see* Geranium spp.

Crateuas, 10, 17, 19, 90

Crescenzi, Pietro, 66-72; biography, 69-70

Crisp, Sir Frank, 70

Crüÿdeboeck, 173-80; contents of, 179; editions of, 180; illustrations, 177-79; other titles, 177; translations of, 178

Cube, Dr. Johann von, 96

Culpeper, Nicholas, 186

Dante, 69

Davalos, Diego Lopez, 243

Degrees defined, 154

De materia medica, 7-15; cited by Simon Januensis, 41; quoted by Macer, 34; quoted by Serapion, 42

Dewes, Gerard, 180

Diana, 24

Diani, Tito, 192

Diaz, Fernando, 209

Diaz, Hernando, 209

Dinckmut, Conrad, 97

Diocles, 17, 19

Dioscorides, Pedanios, 7-15; compared with *Circa instans,* 49; in Apuleius' herbal, 24, 26; in Bartholomaeus Anglicus, 64; lost versions, 40; Mattioli's expansions of, 169-71; Mattioli's obsession with, 164; praised by Dodoens, 178; quoted by Macer, 34; seedlessness of ferns, 134; unknown by Pliny, 19; valerian legend, 211

Dioscorides Renovado, El, 10

Diringer, David, 32

Disibodenberg, 51

Distilier Buch, Das, 113-14, 117; reworked by Lonitzer, 156

Distillation, 117

Doctrine of Signatures, 197-99; condemned, 178

Dodoens, Rembert: biography, 173-75; collaborations, 175,

Dodoens, Rembert (*Continued*)
177; condemns Doctrine of
Signatures, 178; Councilor
Hopper, 174; Malines,
173-74, 179; *Pemptades*,
179-80; tomb, 179; translations of, 178, 180; University
of Leyden, 174-75
Dolphins aid fishermen, 16
Dorsten, Theodore, 156
Dos Libros, 202, 206-9; editions
of, 209; New World plants,
208; posthumous third part,
208; translations of, 209
Drach, Peter, 72
Durante, Castore, 187

Early firearms, 77
Earthquake and plague, 77
Ebers Papyrus, 159-60
Edward VI, 149-50
Egenolph, Christian, 15, 122,
129; artists and block-cutters,
157; heirs of, 157, 162; loses
law-suit, 156-57; plagiariza-
tions, 157; Rösslin's herbal,
156
Ekphrasis, 216
Elizabeth I: befriends Turner,
151-52; Bezoar stone of, 162
Enax, 89
Erfurt, 138
Erigeron, *see Senecio vulgaris*
Escorial, 235, 240
Escrivano, Alonso, 209
Etched illustrations, 213-14

Fabro, Ioanne, 243
Falls Village, Conn., 234
Felix Platter Herbarium, 124
Ferdinard I, 164, 185
Ficalho, Conde de, 206, 209

Fischer, P., 200
Frampton, John, 208-9
Frankfurt, 92, 96, 107, 122, 129,
156, 162, 172, 190, 192, 200
Frankincense, *see Boswellia carteri*
Frederick II, 70
Fuchs, Leonhart: biography,
138, 140; cuts used by Dodoens, 177; "German father
of botany," 51; his illustrators, 145; "masculine" and
"feminine" plants, 138; medical concerns, 137; supervises
illustrations, 143; "sweating
sickness," 138
Füllmaurer, Heinrich, 145
Furter, Michael, 97

Galen, 34, 42, 112
Gargilius Martialis, 34
Garrison, Fielding, 39
Gart der Gesundheit, Der, 89-97;
Arbolayre illustrations, 98,
105; authorship, 96; cites
Pliny, 20; cites Serapion, 44;
contents, 93-94; editions, 97;
Grant Herbier illustrations,
98, 105; *Hortus sanitatis* illustrations, 107; illustrations of,
89-90; plagiarized, 96-97;
prologue, 96
Geranium spp., 56
Gerard, John, 218-26; Barber-
Surgeons Co., 218-20; biography, 218-20; death, 220; errors with illustrations,
224-25; Holborn gardens,
219; illness, 225; influential
connections, 218-19; Norton,
220-22, 224; oversights by,
234; plagiarism by, 223; por-

trait, 219; writing ability, 225-26
Goa, 202, 206, 209
Goodyer, John, 15, 232, 234
Gorizia, 164
Grabadin of Mesue, 37, 44
Graeco-Roman authors, portraits of, 24
Graf, Urs, 112
Grant Herbier, Le, 98-105; and *Circa instans,* 98-99, 101-5; damaged copies, 99; editions, 98, 105; Modena mss., 101, 105; number of chapters, 99, 102; sources, 98, 104-5; two traditions, 99
Grete Herball, 99, 148
Grosse Destillierbuch, 114, 120
Groundsel, *see Senecio vulgaris*
Grüninger, Johann: combats plagiarism, 114; edits Brunschwig's text, 113-14; edition of *Der Gart,* 97, 107; editions of *Distilierbuch,* 113-14, 119; illustrations in *Arbolayre,* 105; illustrations criticized, 114; publisher of Brunschwig, 114
Guaiacum, 239
Guelphs and Ghibellines, 70
Guibert of Gembloux, 52
Gülfferich, Herman, 112
Gulielmus of Pavia, 88
Gunther, Robert T., 15, 26
Gutenberg, Johann, 82

Haller, Albrecht von, 48; erroneously cited, 211
Hamon, Physician to Suleiman the Great, 10
Heaven's Keys, *see Primula vulgaris*

Heidelsheim, 132
Hempseed, *see Cannabis sativa*
Henry VII, 109
Henry VIII, 149
Hentzske, Michael, 186
Herbal of Apuleius, 23-29, 30; Anglo-Saxon translation, 26, 29; diagrammatic illustrations, 81; editions, 29; false attribution, 24; manuscripts, 26, 29; Peleus-Apuleius, 24; Plato-Platearius, 25; Pre-Christian origin, 26-27; various titles, 23
Herball of John Gerard, 218-26; authorship problems, 225; editions, 226; Gerard's contributions, 225-26; illustrations rented, 224; L'Obel's contributions, 224-25; Norton's edition, 220-24, 226; parallels Lyte, 223; potato, 219, 226
Herbario Nuovo, 187-92; alphabetical order, 187; artists, 191; editions, 192; German translation, 190, 192; illustrations, 191-92; Latin verses, 189; number of chapters, 191; polyglot lists, 189
Herbarius latinus, 81, 82-88; aliases, 83-84; cites Serapion, 44; contents, 86-87; editions and translations, 82, 88; false ascription, 84; illustrations, 83; initiates title page, 83; plagiarized, 87; purpose, 83; sample remedies, 87; sources, 87-88
Herbarius zu Teutsch: confused with Herbarius latinus, 84
Herbarum Vivae Eicones, 121-29;

Herbarum Vivae Eicones (Cont.)
editions, 129; German translation, 129; illustrations discovered, 124; quality of illustrations, 121; shortcomings of, 125-27; von Weiditz's contribution, 121-24, 129

Hernandez, Francisco: Aztecs, 236; biography, 235-36, 239-40; *chupire*, 237; disappointments, 240; expenses, 236, 239; lists native names, 237; meets hostility, 235; Mexican hazards, 237; Protomedico, 236; relations with Philip II, 235-36, 239-40

Hertz, Michele, 192

Hildegarde of Bingen: biography, 51-52; lion's heart remedy, 56; natural history, 51; *Physica*, 51-52, 56; practice of medicine, 52, 56; visions, 52

Hippocrates, 34, 63

Hist, J. and C., 88

Histoire des Plantes, 180

Historia naturalis, 16-22, 39; editions and translations, 22; manuscripts, 18, 22; plant sections, 18-19; sources of, 17, 19; statistics of, 17

Historia Stirpium, 137-47; arrangement, 138; colored copies, 145-46; editions, 146-47; illustrations, 145; illustrators, 145; indices, 138; Linnaeus' types, 146; maize illustrated, 145; new species, 146; pictorial editions, 146-47; plant introductions, 146; translations, 146-47; woodcuts sold, 147

Historia of Thurneisser, 181-86; deceit in, 183-85; editions, 186

Hoffman, Nicklaus (Nicolaum), 192, 200

Hohenstaufen, 70

Holland, Philemon, 22

Holy Roman Emperors: Ferdinand I, 164; Maximilian II, 10, 164; 174; Rudolph II, 174

Honoratae, 11

Hortus sanitatis, 106-12; anonymous work, 106; chapters, 106; contents, 111; editions, 107, 111-12; fashions, 109; illustrations, 106-7, 111; index, 108; lodestone legend, 111; prices, 109; source of *Noble Lyfe . . .* , 107-8; sources of, 109; translations, 107, 112

Hudson, Noel, 108

Hunger, F.W.T., 26

Hufflatich, *see Tussilago farfara*

Huss, Matthias, 65

Hymelsluszel, *see Primula vulgaris*

Ibn Sārabiyūn or Sārāfyūn, *see* Serapion

Ibn Sina, *see* Avicenna

Imperato, Ferrante, 194

Ingolstadt, 138

Isidore of Seville, 60, 63, 232; *Etymologiarum*, 62

Isingrin, Michael, 146-47; printer's device, 147

James I, 44, 227

Johannem Allemanum de Medemblick, 15

John of Trevisa, 64
Johnson, Thomas, 227, 234;
edits Gerard, 226
*Joyfull Newes Out of the Newe
Founde Worlde*, 208-9
Juliana Anicia, 11; Codex,
10-11, 15

Kandel, David: adapts from
Brunfels, 134; adapts from
Fuchs, 134, 146; editions il-
lustrated by, 136; original
contributions, 134
Kempffer, Matthew, 162
Klebs, Arnold, 49-50, 90, 97
Kleine Destillierbuch, 114; En-
glish translation, 119
Kreüter Buch of J. Bock, 130-36;
ecology, 133-34; editions,
136; innovations, 130, 132;
Latin translation, 134;
phytography, 132; picture
sources, 134
Kuilenberg, 88
Kyber, David: death of, 134;
Latin translation, 134, 136

Latomus, Sigismund, 162
Le Caron, Pierre, 105
Lechler, Martin, 162
Leclerc, Lucien, 42
L'Ecluse, Charles, *see* Clusius
Lelamar, John, 30
Leno, Francesco de, 88
Le Noir, Philippe, 112
Leo Africanus, 37
Leon, Dr. Nicolas, 244
Leyden, 174-75, 179
Libellus de re herbaria novus, 148
Liber aggregatus of Serapion, 44,
48-50

Liber de arte distillandi . . . .,
113, 117; date of 1st edition,
119
Liberale, Giorgio, 167
Licinius Bassus, 8
Lignamine, Philip de, 26, 29
Linnaeus, Carolus: uses Fuchs
illustrations, 146
Linné, Carl, *see* Linnaeus,
Carolus
Lisbon, 202, 206, 209
L'Obel, Matthias: aids Gerard
224-25; botanical work, 173,
175, 177; system substituted,
223
Lodestone, 111
Loe, Henry, 180
Loe, Jan vander, 177, 180
Loeb Classical Library, 22
London, 150, 155, 209, 219,
226-27, 234; flora of Mid-
dlesex, 232; near famine, 225
London Dispensatory: cites
Serapion, 44
London Pharmacopeia: cites
Mesue, 44
Lonitzer, Adam: biography,
157; edits herbal, 156;
Egenolph's son-in-law, 157;
inherits from Egenolph, 157
Lonitzer's *Kreütterbuch*, 156-62;
ancient lore, 159-60; edi-
tions, 162; Fuchs's criticism,
158; incorporates
Brunschwig, 156, 158; long
life of, 157; originality lack-
ing, 156; perpetuates myths,
160-61; pirated illustrations,
156; varying versions, 157
Louvain, 87-88
Lübeck, 97
Lyons, 65, 98, 147, 172, 209

Lyte, Henry, 178, 180, 221, 223, 225

Macer Floridus' *De viribus herbarum*, 30-35; authorship, 30-32; author's origin, 32-33; editions, 35; first printed herbal, 39; manuscripts of, 32, 35; rarely discussed, 32; sources, 34; spurious sections, 32; total chapters, 32; use of verse, 32, 34
Madrid, 240-43
Madurensis, 24
Magdeburg, 59
Mainz, 51, 82-83, 88, 92, 96, 97, 106, 109, 111, 128, 157
Malines, 173-74, 179; destroyed, 174
Mandragora officinalis, 64, 200
Mandrake, *see Mandragora officinalis*
Manuscript rentals, 92
Manutius, Aldus, 15
Markham, Sir Clements R., 209
Māsawaih al-Māradīnī, *see* Mesue
Mascardi, J., 243
Mascardi, V., 243
Materia medica: Aztec system, 236; Dioscorides', 7-15; exotic sources, 202; in Parkinson's *Theatrum*, 228; Macer imitated, 189; revision needed, 212; set apart, 230
Mattioli, Pier Andrea, 163-71; at Goritzia, 164; at Rome, 163; at Trent, 164, 171; authority on Dioscorides, 164; biography, 163-64; children, 164; controversies, 168; Court physician, 164, 166;

death, 164, 171; education, 163; expansive commentaries, 169-71; experiments with criminals, 171; faulty methods, 168; his mottoes, 171; list for dispute, 168; marriages, 164; retirement, 164, 174
Maximilian II, 10, 182, 185
Mayer, Albrecht, 145
Mechlin, *see* Malines
Medieval beliefs, 57
Melancholy prevented by coal, 89
Melantrich, Georgen, 172
Mesue the Elder: note, 36
Mesue the Younger (Pseudo-Mesue), 36-39, 44; works of, 37, 39, 44
Meteor, 77
Metlinger, Pierre, 105
Mexico City, 244
Meydenbach, Jacob, 106-7, 111
Meyer, Ernst, 17, 48-49, 178
Meyerpeck, Wolfgang, 167
Mierdman, Steven, 155
Milan, 35, 44
Misenum, 20
Modena, 101, 105
Monardes, Nicolas, 202, 206-9; credulity, 207-8; editions, 209; New World unvisited, 206; other writings, 208
Monkshood, *see Aconitum napellus*
Montecorvo, 240
Morelia, 244
Moretus, Balthasar and Johannes, 180
Munting, Abraham, 199
Mushroom poisoning, 74-75
Myristica fragrans, 57, 205

Names of Herbes, 148

Naples, 35, 193-94, 200, 210, 217, 243

National Library of Austria, 10

Natural History of Pliny, *see Naturalis historiae*

Naturalis historiae of Pliny, 16-22, 39; editions, 22; English translations, 22; manuscripts, 22

Natural Magick of G.B. Porta, 199

Natura rerum, 60, 74

Nero, 8, 20

New Herball of Wm. Turner, 148-55; complete herbal, 152, 155; editions, 150, 152, 155; defines degrees, 154-55; herbal banned, 151; local flora recognized, 152; native plants, 152

Nicholas of Salerno, 48

Nievve Herball, 178, 180

Nissen, Claus, 26, 49, 97, 159

Norsino, Leonardo, 191

Norton, John, 220-24, 226

Nutmeg, *see Myristica fragrans*

Odo, Bishop of Meung, 30-32

Opera Salernitana 'Circa instans' . . . , 105

Opium: remedy for overdose, 153

Opus ruralium commodorum, 66-72; composition of, 70; contents, 67; editions, 66, 72; herbal section, 67; manuscripts, 66, 72; sources, 66, 68-69; translations, 70

Oribasius, 34

Orta, Garcia da: biography, 202; linguistic ability, 203; variant names, 209

Ortega, Casimir Gomez, 243

Otiosi, 194

Oxford, 59, 65

Paradisi in Sole . . . , 228

Parasole, Isabella, 191

Paris, 59-60, 73, 77, 88, 92, 98, 105, 107, 112, 147

Parkinson, John: associates, 227, 234; biography, 227-28; botanical contributions, 232, 234; honors, 227; medieval outlook, 228-29; royal patrons, 227-28

Passau, 88

Peleus, 24

Pembroke College, 149

Pemptades of Dodoens, 177-80, 221

Petri, Johann, 88

Pezzanam, Nicolaum, 172

Pfeiffer, Franz, 79

Philip II of Spain, 174, 235-36, 239-40

Phytobasanos, 210-17; defined, 210; editions, 217; number of plates, 217

Phytognomonica, 193-200; editions, 200; poisoned elephants, 193-94; title translated, 199

Planco, Iano, 217

Plantin, Christophe, 177-80, 209

Plantin Press, 206, 209; artists at, 178-79; colorists at, 146; L'Obel published, 177; low pay at, 178

Platearius, Matthaeus: Cantimpré adapts, 74; *Circa in-*

268

Platearius, Matthaeus (*Cont.*) *stans*, 46; cited by Bartholomaeus, 63-64; Crescenzi's use of, 68-69; error in Apuleius, 25; in *Le Grant Herbier*, 104; neglect of, 48-49; quoted, 48; teacher-physician, 46

Plato, 25

Pliny (Caius Plinius Secundus), 16-22, 49, 60, 63, 69, 109, 137; biography, 20-21; cited in herbals, 20; Cousteau, 16; criticized, 17; Dioscorides ignored, 19; Erigeron remedy, 34; his data, 17; in Apuleius, 26; in Macer, 34; Spanish translation, 239-40

Polyeuktos, 11

Pompeii, 20

Porta, Giambattista: astrologist, 196; biography, 193-94; brother, 194; Doctrine of Signatures, 197-99; exact sciences, 194; founds Otiosi, 194; Lincei, 194; mandrake, 200; *Natural Magick*, 199

Potato: earliest depiction, 219, 226

Prague, 164, 172

Primrose, *see Primula vulgaris*

Primula vulgaris, 56

Printed illustrations: first botanical, 81; first zoological, 81

Pritzel, G.A., 48, 81

Proprietatibus Rerum, 59-65; authorities used, 64; contents, 62; editions, 60, 65; errors, 63; herbal section, 63-64; model for, 62; rationale of, 62-63; rival works, 60; rose, 64-65; time system, 65

Prüss, Johann, 107, 111-12

Quincy, John, 10, 44

Rainbow, white, 77

Rangoni (Tommaso Gianotti), 199

Ratisbon, 73-74, 81

Ray, John, 234

Recchi, Dr. Nardo Antonio, 240, 242-43

Regimen Salernitanum, 34

Register, early use of, 215

Rerum Medicarum . . . of Hernandez, 235-44; Aztec aid, 236; destroyed, 240; editions, 243; ethnobotany, 236-37; extracts, 240; guaiacum, 239; manuscripts, 239-40, 242-43; notable items, 238-39; paper, 239; publication of, 240, 242-43

Rihel, Josias, 136

Rihel, Wendel, 136

Robert Grosseteste, 59

Rome, 187, 192, 194, 243; sack of, 163

Rose, 57, 64-65

Rösslin, Eucharius, 156-57

Rouen, 40, 200

Ruano, Dr., 204-5

Rubia tinctorum, 42

Rupertsberg, 52

Ruppel, Berthold, 60, 65

Sachs, Julius, 124

St. Gall, 28

Salernitan illustrations, 82, 90

Salernitans, 33, 48

Salerno, 25, 52, 69; Platearii of, 46; School of, 33, 46, 48

Salviani, Horatio, 200

Saponaria officinalis, 48

Sarton, George, 37, 49, 60, 101

Saxony, 59

Schoeffer, Peter, 82-83, 86-90, 92, 96-97; branch offices, 92, 96; Fust, 83; Gutenberg, 82; illustration improved, 89-90; useful indices, 92-93

Schoensperger, Hanns, 97

Schoensperger, Johann, 96, 97, 107, 114

Schott, Johann, 58, 122, 129; sues Egenolph, 156

Schroeder, Johann, 199

Schussler, Johann, 72

Scoti, Octaviani, 50

Scriptores Rei Rusticae, 66

Scriptoria, 90; fees paid in, 92

Sebizius, Melchior, 136

Secres de Salerne, 101, 103-5

Senation, *see Senecio vulgaris*

Senecio vulgaris, 34

Serapion, 36, 40-44, 49-50; citations of, 44; editions, 44; Hebrew manuscript, 42; Simon Januensis, 40, 42

Serapion Senior: note, 36

Sessa, Melchior, 22

Seville, 206, 208-9, 236

Sexti Platonici Papyrensis, 24

Sextius Niger, 19

Siena, 163

Simon Januensis (Simon of Genoa), 40, 42

Simples: defined, 45-46; problems of, 46

Singer, Charles, 26, 29

Soapwort, *see Saponaria officinalis*

Speckle, Veit Rudolph, 145

Speier, 87-88

Speyer, 72

Spira, Johann, 22

Stabiae, 20

Starkenstein Mss., 49-50

Stationers (Stationarii), 90, 92

Still-room, 119

Storcksnabel, *see Geranium spp.*

Strassburg, 97, 107, 109, 111-12, 114, 119-20, 128-29, 132, 136, 156, 181, 185

Strucium, *see Saponaria officinalis*

Tacuinis, Joannes, 112

Tarsus, 8

Terrentio, Ioanne, 243

Theatrum Botanicum, 227-34; botanical order, 230; completeness of, 228; dedication of, 228; reprint, 234; statistics of, 227; synonyms in, 232

Theophrastus, 8, 126, 130, 136, 212

Thomas de Cantimpré, 60, 73-74

Thorndike, Lynn, 49

Thure, *see Boswellia carteri*

Thurneisser, Leonhard, 181-85; astrology and alchemy, 181-85; biography, 181-82; correspondents, 182; death of, 182; plant classification, 185

Toothache remedy, 34

Touchstone, 210

Tradescant, John, 227, 234

Trent, 163-64, 171
Trotula (Dame Trot), 46
Tubingen, 138
Tumor remedy, 34
Turner, William: banished, 149-51; biography, 149-52; books destroyed, 150-51; botanical innovations, 152; death, 152; defines degrees, 154-55; nonconformity, 149, 152; plant names, 148-49; retires, 152; royalty, 149-52; theology, 149, 152; titles, 149; travels, 149
Tussilago farfara, 56

Uffenbachium, Petrum, 192
Ulm, 97, 162
Uroscopy, 94-96, 106, 111-12

Valeriana officinalis: aid for epilepsy, 211
Valgrisio, Vincentio, 44, 164, 166, 172
Varnhagen, F.A. de, 209
Vegetable Lamb, 229-30
Veldener, Jan, 88
Venice, 15, 22, 44, 50, 88, 109, 112, 163-64, 166, 171-72, 192, 199, 209

Verard, Antoine, 107, 112
Vespasian, 20
Vesuvius, 20
Vicenza, 88
Vienna, 10, 15, 35, 50, 73-74, 79, 164, 174
Villa d'Olma, 70, 72
Vincent of Beauvais, 57, 60, 73, 88; *Speculum majus . . . ,* 88

Wagner, Matthew, 162
Wechel, J., 200
Weiditz, Hans von, 129; artistry, 121; botanical grasp, 122-24; Egenolph, 157; originals, 124
Wemding, 138
Witchcraft, 34
Wolffischen, Joseph, 162
Women of Salerno, 48, 69
Wound remedy, 34

Ximenez, Fray Francisco, 242-44

Zarotus, Antonius, 35, 44
Zea mays: first illustration, 145
Zweibrucken, 132